CHRIS YUILL, IAIN CRINSON AND EILIDH DUNCAN

Key Concepts in
Health Studies

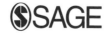

Los Angeles | London | New Delhi
Singapore | Washington DC

First published 2010

SAGE Publications Ltd
1 Oliver's Yard
55 City Road
London EC1Y 1S
SAGE Publications Inc.
2455 Teller Road
Thousand Oaks, California 91320

SAGE Publications India Pvt Ltd
B 1/I 1 Mohan Cooperative Industrial Area
Mathura Road, New Delhi 110 044
India

SAGE Publications Asia-Pacific Pte Ltd
33 Pekin Street #02-01
Far East Square
Singapore 048763

British Library Cataloguing in Publication data

A catalogue record for this book is available from the
British Library

ISBN978-1-84860-673-9
ISBN978-1-84860-674-6

Library of Congress Control Number Available

Typeset by C&M Digitals (P) Ltd, Chennai, India
Printed in Great Britain by CPI Antony Rowe, Chippenham, Wiltshire
Printed on paper from sustainable resources

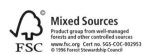

Key Concepts in
Health Studies

contents

contents

v

key concepts in
health studies

notes on the text

At the end of each entry, the initials of the author are shown:

Iain Crinson   I. C.
Eilidh Duncan   E. D.
Chris Yuill   C. Y.

Many concepts contain cross-references in bold guiding readers to related concepts.

notes on the authors

Chris Yuill is a lecturer in the sociology of health at Robert Gordon University, Aberdeen. He is the author of 'Understanding the Sociology of Health: A Sociological Introduction' (2008) London, SAGE, and his academic interests lie in the sociology of health inequalities.

Iain Crinson is senior lecturer in the sociology of health and health policy at St George's, University of London. He is the author of 'Health Policy; A Critical Perspective' (2009) London, SAGE, and his academic interests lie in the sociology of the healthcare professions, inequalities in health, and the impact of information technology within the NHS.

Eilidh Duncan is a lecturer in psychology at Robert Gordon University, Aberdeen. She graduated with a BSc (Hons) in Psychology from the University of Glasgow, and gained an MSc in Health Psychology from the University of Stirling. Eilidh is currently completing a PhD from Robert Gordon University investigating alcohol and nicotine use during pregnancy and is working towards chartership as a Health Psychologist.

key concepts in
health studies

Introduction

For most people, health is about what you eat and how much exercise you take, and if something goes wrong there's always the medical profession there to patch you up and get you back to what you were doing previously. Health Studies seeks to go beyond this narrow perception of health. Health Studies is animated by an understanding that health is much more than 'blood and bones', or only intelligible through the workings and ideas of mainstream medicine. The idea of 'health' emerges out of an array of diverse social processes and influences, many of these processes operating at levels beyond the physical body with which we experience life in all its states, good or bad. Culture, politics, ethics, emotions, our spiritual selves, and our social and individual perceptions of the world all contribute to what makes us healthy or not.

The great strength of Health Studies as a field of academic study is that it is built on the contributions of many disciplines. It draws on sociology, psychology, social policy, social epidemiology, ethics, anthropology and biology in an attempt to build the big picture of health. Each discipline possesses its particular strengths in contributing to an overall understanding of health. For example, sociology explores social processes and structures, and so aids an understanding of how our social class, our gender or our ethnicity influence and shape our health. Psychology investigates the psychological factors that may determine health, such as personality, stress and beliefs, and seeks to explain the thought processes that are fundamental to health behaviour. And social policy provides insights into how governments, charities and private companies structure their services and the thinking behind why they do so.

This textbook should be seen as part of the journey that you are now undertaking in exploring health in its fullest, richest and deepest sense. On offer here is a selection of key concepts that should ease that process. It will help you get to grips with a new way of thinking about the world by providing short summaries of the main concepts that you will encounter. Each entry on a key concept opens with a very brief definition of its main features before going on to outline the main issues and debates that the concept has generated. As such, you can build a firm basis on which to further discuss and read more on each concept.

This textbook book is not an end in itself. The outlines of the key assumptions of concepts widely utilized within Health Studies are presented, and some context for their application is also provided, However, applying these concepts to further understanding of real-world health issues also requires students to engage in more in-depth reading; hence the suggestions for further reading at the close of most entries. By pursuing these suggestions, your knowledge both of a concept and of Health Studies overall will be greatly enriched, allowing you to be more confident in your studies, in doing well in your assessments and possibly learning and understanding more about what shapes your health and the health of other people around you.

This book is structured into six parts, each of which deals with a specific issue within Health Studies, building from very general philosophical approaches before moving on to concepts that relate to practice and the structuring of health services.

Part 1 surveys on various concepts that attempt to capture and *define health*. Here, you can contrast different models of health that influence and inform how notions of health are constructed and maintained within society. Key here are the fundamentally different outlooks of the biomedical and social models of health. These tensions inform many of the other concepts described in the book, and are a central concern of Health Studies. This section provides an awareness of what makes Health Studies distinct from other approaches to an understanding of health and what insights Health Studies have to offer.

Part 2 centres on the *human life course* and outlines a range of concepts which relate to the 'transitions' and 'trajectories' that occur in everyone's lives. Evident here is how what may seem like an intrinsically biological process, that of growing from infancy to adulthood and on to old age before dying, is in practice bound up with a variety of social, cultural and psychological processes. From infancy on, through childhood and beyond, society and culture are always present, creating and conditioning everyday experiences, identity and health.

Part 3 turns to the notion of *health protection*. This is a term now widely used to describe national and international strategies to reduce threats to the health of populations (in the UK, for example, the Health Protection Agency is responsible for identifying and responding to all sorts of environmental threats and hazards, and improving our understanding and knowledge of these threats). This section looks at these issues in terms of health inequalities and global health risks, and the strategies deployed to counter these outcomes, such as public health interventions and health promotion initiatives.

In Part 4 we turn our attention to *health beliefs and health behaviour*. The concepts explored in this section seek to explain and contextualize the ways in which ordinary people perceive, understand and are motivated (or otherwise) about their health.

People actively interpret and filter messages and understandings of health through social, personal and cultural traditions and experiences. Again, this observation informs us about the subtleties of health and the rich variety of meanings attached to health in wider society. As human beings we remain bounded by our physical bodies, and to that extent our body both strongly shapes our self-identity and self-conceptions, and vice versa. The notion of the 'self', while being clearly different from the body, is nevertheless frequently experienced as one and the same thing. This interconnectivity between biology, the social and the psychological is explored in a variety of ways in this section.

In Part 5 we consider a vital aspect of *the lived experience of health and illness*. People experience being healthy or ill in a variety of ways. Research has identified that the functional medical aspects of being ill, attending a clinic, taking medication or following a treatment regimen, for example, are just one element of the experience of health and illness. How one maintains a sense of self and how one copes with the emotional tasks associated with pain and suffering can be just as important, if not more so, than medical concerns.

The book concludes with a final section exploring the forms of *health care provision* in all its aspects. Rightly or wrongly, most people perceive the health care system as the key tangible representation of health management within a society reflected in the support the public gives to these services and the continuing financial commitment of government. However, as has been observed many times, health care systems have little to do with health, rather, their function is to manage illness. These systems are explored in this section from the perspective of those who work within them, from the service users' perspective, and from the perspective of those who until recently have been ignored, excluded from or damaged by the health care system. Challenges to existing mechanisms of health care are also explored through the concepts of 'governance' and 'consumerism'.

We trust that you find the book useful and stimulating and that you come away after reading it knowing more about the subject that you are studying. If there is one overall message that this book is trying to communicate, it is that health exists in many interweaving dimensions, some obvious and apparent, others subtle and hidden. Health is about the body, the biological, but that is just one element of the many different relationships, processes and factors that ultimately constitute health.

3

Think too about the social, the psychological, the ethical, the spiritual, the cultural and many other elements that frame, influence, shape and make sense of health.

Chris Yuill, Iain Crinson and Eilidh Duncan

key concepts in
health studies

Part 1
Defining Health

The biomedical model of health

The medical, or as it has more properly become known, the 'biomedical' or 'scientific' model, draws upon biochemical explanations of ill health as the basis for treatment and intervention, as opposed to the focus of other forms of non-allopathic medicine (see **Alternative or complementary medicine**).

Many sociologists and others have for sometime argued that despite the undoubted achievements of biomedical interventions in the management of particular forms of illness (but also see **Medicalization**), and the very real effects of biological mechanisms in illness, the practice of biomedicine remains rooted in a knowledge base that is not as empirically-bound as biomedical scientists would have us believe. However, to the extent that biomedical knowledge is concerned to categorize and manipulate an understanding of biological mechanisms in order to contextualize the reality of the human illness, it is a process of knowledge construction which implicitly involves cultural and social assumptions as well as drawing upon a biological base of understanding (Lock, 1988).

The continuing dominance of the biomedical model or paradigm within modern health care systems is reflected in the day-to-day rational–scientific practices associated with the work of doctors in the hospital or clinic. For Foucault (1973) and those influenced by a relational conceptualization of power, these everyday clinical practices have contributed to the (social) construction and reproduction of what is termed the 'biomedical discourse'. A 'discourse' being the means through which we have come to know, understand and respond to aspects of our lives; in this case, our health and illness. Studies in the history of medicine have demonstrated the ways in which this biomedical discourse has been shaped not only by an emergent scientific understanding of the biological mechanisms of the human body, but also by other social, economic and cultural developments.

For example, Jewson's (1976) classic work on the development and production of medical knowledge identified a series of what he termed 'medical cosmologies', or ways of seeing the contribution of medicine to the diagnosis and treatment of the sick. Jewson drew on these 'cosmologies' to describe the ways in which developments in medicine have historically been intimately linked with the sets of social relations and dominant ideas existing within society at the time. The *person-orientated* cosmology was seen as existing prior to industrialization and the 'Age of Enlightenment'. This approach to the practice of medicine required the physician to recognize the patient as a holistic entity, and where medical judgement was to be made in terms of the personal attributes of the sick person (if they were not, then the physician would lose the business!).

The early development of hospital-based medicine in the late eighteenth century is seen as being associated with the broader social changes occurring within British society at that time. The rise, that is, of capitalist forms of production, industrialization, the growth of towns and cities, and the increasing dominance of scientific knowledge and explanation. The emergence of a specialist scientific medical knowledge reflects the historical period in which the doctor–patient balance of power begins to change, and is described as an *object-orientated* cosmology. At this time the medical profession was becoming less dependent upon patronage of rich patients, and the control of medical knowledge began to pass from the patient to the clinician. Hospitals now became training centres for the new profession of medicine and sites for scientific research. The late nineteenth century witnessed the emergence of Jewson's third medical cosmology, that of *laboratory medicine*. Here, the patient as the object of medical practice moves out of the frame, and disease becomes a 'physio-chemical process'. This practice is characterized by the emergence of what Foucault (1973) termed the new 'clinical gaze', reflecting the changing social relationship of power between doctors and their patients.

The main methodological and philosophical assumptions of some of the key components of the biomedical model or 'discourse' are set out and explored below:

- A knowledge base that draws in large part upon a *positivist* methodology. Positivism is the philosophical position that science can only examine what is observable and measurable. Knowledge of anything beyond that is deemed to be impossible. It follows then that only observable signs and symptoms can lead to a medical 'diagnosis', all 'real' disease has to have measurable biological causal mechanisms. This approach has, in the past, frequently led to the marginalization and neglect of social and psychological factors in ill health.
- Health defined as the absence of any biological *abnormality* or change. Therefore 'disease' as its obverse is conceived as predominantly a

biological state associated with the malfunctioning of human biological systems. This is essentially a biologically reductionist view in that all forms of illness are seen as causally related to specific biochemical mechanisms.

- The (ontological) separation of the *mind and body*. This philosophical notion derives from the work of the seventeenth-century philosopher René Descartes, who distinguished between the *res cogitans* and the *res extensa*. The former referred to the soul or mind and was said to be essentially 'a thing which thinks', while the latter referred to the material stuff of the body. The latter is much more amenable to observation and measurement, and so enabled the emergence of modern bioscience and the practice of biomedicine (Bracken and Thomas, 2002). The legacy of this 'Cartesian split' within biomedicine has been a rejection of any possible connection between the mind or psyche and physicality. This distinction is now beginning to be addressed by more recent developments in neuroscience.

- The *reification* (i.e. to make an essentially abstract idea into something concrete or 'natural') of disease categories. The specific notion of disease that we all understand today (as a discrete set of pathological processes that can be isolated and located with body organs and tissues) first appeared with the emergence of modern medicine. The process of constructing diseases categories bundled together observed and measurable 'deviations' from the 'normal' functioning of the body (often distinguishing between those localized to specific organs and those deemed to be more general or systemic within the body), was crucial to the (social) construction of a body of clinical knowledge with which to train doctors and develop biomedical interventions. Drawing distinctions between the pathological effects of different diseases enabled a set of nosological (classificatory) tables to be drawn up. Yet, from the very beginning of modern medicine, the process of disease classification was not solely based on bioscientific knowledge of the 'natural' and the 'pathological'. There is an extensive literature which has documented, for example, the ways in which women were frequently 'diagnosed' as suffering from 'hysteria' when their behaviour appeared to fall outside particular social norms. This example and many others reflect the social, political and cultural assumptions surrounding the process of disease classification. The process of disease classification is ongoing, with the *International Classification of Diseases* (ICD) now in its 10th edition (for a history of the development of the ICD, see WHO, 2008). This history demonstrates the contested and often uncertain nature of the practice of disease classification that the process of reifying disease would deny.

- The doctrine of *specific aetiology*. This is the oversimplified notion that draws on the positivist methodology (described above) that pathologies have single linear causality, i.e. a TB bacillus invades the 'host' (individual) bringing about the development of a particular form of tuberculosis (Comaroff, 1982). In practice, this doctrine has served to limit the understanding of the environmental factors that make individuals and social groups more susceptible to disease.

However, drawing attention to the biomedical 'discourse' does not constitute the case for arguing that the whole edifice of biomedicine is purely a social construction as some commentators would claim. What it does do is to question the claim to scientific rigour of all biomedical and clinical practice. Indeed, the practice of Medicine is sometime described as an 'Art' by clinicians themselves. What is being referred to here is the practice of making a diagnosis based on experience and the synthesis of a series of clinical 'facts' and 'data' about an individual patient from a variety of sources. The attempt is then made to connect this often incomplete and context-specific knowledge to a 'textbook' disease classification which is not always a systemic process; hence the notion of medical practice as an 'art' (Berg, 1992).

REFERENCES

Berg, M. (1992) 'The construction of medical disposals', *Sociology of Health and Illness*, 14(2): 151–81.

Bracken, P. and Thomas, P. (2002) 'Time to move beyond the mind–body split', *British Medical Journal*, 325: 1433–4.

Comaroff, J. (1982) 'Medicine, symbol and ideology', in P. Wright and A. Treacher (eds), *The Problem of Medical Knowledge: Examining the Social Construction of Medicine*. Edinburgh: University of Edinburgh Press.

Foucault, M. (1973) *The Birth of the Clinic: An Archaeology of Medical Perception*. London: Tavistock.

Jewson, N. (1976) 'The disappearance of the sick man from medical cosmology 1770–1870', *Sociology*, 10: 225–44.

Lock, M. (1988) *Biomedicine Examined*. London: Kluwer Academic Publishers.

WHO (World Health Organization) (2008) *International Classification of Diseases: History of ICD*. Available at: http://www.who.int/classifications/icd/en/History OfICD. pdf (accessed April 2009).

I. C.

The social model of health

The social model of health offers a distinctive and holistic definition and understanding of health that moves beyond the limitations and reductionism associated with the medical model of health. Health, according to the social model, is not a state of being solely under the domain of the medical profession, nor is health and disease only made intelligible by findings of medical science. Rather, a perspective of health is realized that embraces all aspects of human experience and places health fully in the dynamic interplay of social structures and embodied human agency. Such an approach in understanding health is crucial for Health Studies as it allows a wider understanding of health, one that accords with the multidisciplinary basis of the Health Studies approach and provides an excellent conceptual vantage point for the study of health.

The key elements of the social model of health are identified and outlined below. Many of the themes, such as the role of wider social and psychological elements, are encountered throughout this textbook and in many respects this entry provides a condensed overview of the ideas that animate Health Studies.

Individual health is enabled or inhibited by social context. A common lay perception of health, and one that is frequently found in media representations, is that what makes people healthy or ill is down to their own choices. People choose, for example, to eat the 'wrong' sort of high-fat sugary foods, or choose not to diet regularly or choose to engage in risk activities such as smoking. While the power and influence of human agency (ability to make decisions) cannot be ignored, only about a third of poor health can be explained by the choices people make. To further an understanding of health choices it is important to consider that people have to make sense of their lives as conditioned by the specific context in which they find themselves and in which they exercise that agency. Social distinctions such as class, gender and ethnicity also differentially shape the experience of these social contexts and it is to these that we must turn in order to have a fuller social conceptualization of health.

Where someone is socially 'located' allows (or denies) access to certain resources, such as the ability to participate in certain power relationships or to emotionally experience life in a certain way. Social class provides a useful example here. On average, both men and women from social class five live shorter lives than their counterparts in social class one (approximately, 7.5 years for men and 5 for women); they will also experience more life-limiting illness, be exposed to greater chances of disability and will age quicker overall. The reasons for the variance between social classes can be found in how class shapes people's lives. Different social classes have access to better or worse material resources (good housing, for example) and to how much control and power they can exert over their lives. The work of Marmot (2005) indicates that those with more control over their lives tend to have healthier lives than those with low control. How much control one can effect is, in turn, strongly related to social class.

The body is simultaneously social, psychological and biological. The social model of health understands that the human body is much more than simply biology, physiology and anatomy. Instead, the human body is perceived as being bound up in and emerging from many different relationships involving biological, social, psychological, cultural and individual processes. One important process is that of identity. It is both through and with the body that self-identity is enacted and performed. Daily routines attest to this practice with the styling of hair, the selection of particular clothes or the pursuit of the 'perfect' toned gym body. The use of the body to display identity is heightened in consumer societies where appearance can be everything. That sense of identity can be challenged and questioned by the onset of chronic illness, for example. Bury (1991) in his sociological work on chronic illness identifies how chronic illness disrupts an individual's biography triggering a re-evaluation of sense of self.

Health is cultural. The ways in which health is perceived and the experiences of disease and illness are expressed vary by culture. Health and healing have long been important aspects of human existence and all cultures have developed particular norms by which to express the changes that illness brings to their state of being. For example, South Asian people express mental distress using physical metaphors referring to pains in the body as opposed to deploying emotional metaphors (Fenton and Charlsey, 2000). As always when discussing culture, care must be taken not to imply that cultural differences in expressing and perceiving health and illness belong only to 'ethnic minority' groups. Within 'ethnic majority' groups too there are varied traditions of relating the experiences of being unwell. Williams's (1983, 1990) research in the North-East of Scotland among older people illustrates this point. He found that the particularly strong variant of Protestantism that informs the local culture lead to a stoical approach to illness. People who were ill were expected to carry on without complaining or drawing attention to their discomfort.

Culture can also exist in the 'sub-cultures' of the office and sports team. Roderick's (2006) research explored the contradictions found among professional footballers on experiencing pain. Given that they were injured, the next logical step would have been to report the injury, but that might have lost them their place on the squad. The players would consequently endure high levels of pain and injury. By doing so, this could exacerbate the injury, thus jeopardizing future performance and their place on the team. This mode of behaviour may seem illogical but is perfectly consistent with the (masculine) culture of the team in not admitting to pain.

Biomedicine and medical science is something – but not everything. There can be a temptation to 'write off' all that biomedicine and medical science purports to do given the criticisms that are levelled against it. Medical science can be upbraided for being biological reductionism, technological determinism and overstating its efficacy. Many of these criticisms are perfectly valid but one should avoid replacing a 'medical imperialism' with a 'social science imperialism'. Simon J. Williams (2001) warns that sometimes social science perspectives can present a caricature of biomedicine to the extent that no medic would recognize the medical model that they are said to be practising. He also points out that medical science does exhibit many strengths, which are unfortunately often ignored by social scientists.

Health is political. Health is not separate from other spheres of society. Political ideology strongly influences the funding and organization of health services, for example. That is why the United States and the United Kingdom have such different health care systems. In the USA, free-market ideology is more dominant than the social-democratic ideology of the UK. Hence in America health care is much more privatized, with the individual having to make their own arrangements through private health insurance, as opposed to the British state-run, public sector National Health Service.

Other voices matter – In terms of understanding, interpreting and experiencing health and illness, the social model acknowledges other viewpoints, knowledges and discourses beyond the medical profession. Lay people possess knowledge at a 'folk', lay and even expert level. Often lay knowledges of health are informed by culture and personal biography. For many people with a chronic illness, for instance, maintaining and constructing a narrative that provides a sense of self and identity is just as, if not more than, important than medical discourses about their condition.

Overall, the social model of health invites us to adopt a deeper and far-ranging perspective and understanding of health. The lessons from biomedicine and medical science are important but health is much more than simply referring to 'blood-and-bones' and seeing it managed in a hospital or physician context. Health, and what makes people healthy, can only be fully understood by exploring the myriad of interactions and influences that emerge out of the complexities of human experience and the various inter-relationships of the mind, body and society.

REFERENCES AND FURTHER READING

Bury, M. (1991) 'The sociology of chronic illness: a review of research and prospects', *Sociology of Health and Illness*, 13(4): 451–68.

Fenton, S. and Charsley, K. (2000) 'Epidemiology and sociology as incommensurate games: accounts from the study of health and ethnicity', *Health*, 4(4): 403–25.

Marmot, M. (2005) 'Social determinants of health inequalities', *The Lancet*, 2365: 1099–2004.

Roderick, M. J. (2006) 'Adding insult to injury: workplace injury in English professional football', *Sociology of Health and Illness*, 28(1): 76–97.

Williams, R. G. A. (1983) 'Concepts of health: an analysis of lay logic', *Sociology*, 17: 185–205.

Williams, R. G. A. (1990) *A Protestant Legacy: Attitudes to Death and Illness Among Older Aberdonians*. Oxford: Clarendon Press.

Williams, S. J. (2001) 'Sociological imperialism and the profession of medicine revisited: where are we now?', *Sociology of Health and Illness*, 23(2): 135–58.

C. Y.

The social and medical models of disability

The medical model of disability locates disability within the individual, leading to the dependence of the 'disabled' upon health and social care professionals for any improvements in their daily lives. Alternatively, the social model of disability focuses on disability as being located in society rather than the individual. Such 'disabling societies' create negative attitudes and prejudice for those with physical and psychological impairments.

The World Health Organization (WHO) estimates that there are approximately 19 million people in the world with a severe disability. Of this, the vast majority of people with a disability (80 per cent) are to be found in low-income countries. In the higher-income countries, disability is also a common feature in those societies (WHO, 2004). Somewhere near 1-in-6 people have a life-limiting illness in the United Kingdom with the greatest concentrations of people reporting life-limiting illnesses being found in people with routine jobs (15 per cent) and those who had never worked or were unemployed (37 per cent) (National Statistics, 2006). What is also notable about disability is that everyone can experience disability at some point in their life. This change can occur as a result of accidents, illness or becoming older. Disabled people are therefore not a 'fixed' group of people, but highly heterogeneous and individual with different forms of impairment and with different social challenges.

Before outlining the various models of disability in greater depth, it is important to consider terminology and the language used to describe and refer to disabled people. Doing so is not some pedantic exercise in what is often pejoratively dismissed as 'political correctness'. Rather, the language that is used reflects very real and very deep power structures and inferences about the status of people with disabilities in society. In the past, terms such as 'cripple' or 'handicapped' were often deployed to describe people with some form of mainly physical 'difference' that did not match up to social expectations of what an ideal or acceptable body should be. The effect these words have is to diminish the social status and humanity of someone with a disability. That is why terms such as 'disabled person' or 'person with a disability' are not just *preferable* but *essential* to use.

It is also important to conceptualize disability correctly. Doing so has great implications both for health professionals in how they interact with disabled people and for society as a whole in how it frames social policies and allocates resources. A useful way to think about conceptualizing disability can be explored when comparing and contrasting the medical and social models of disability. These are two fundamentally different perspectives that lead to different forms of professional–client interactions and social provision. The two main underlying differences to note between the two models are: (1) the location or cause of disability; and (2) whether or not to assign agency over their lives and affairs to disabled people.

The medical model, as the name suggests, understands disability in the context of the biological and physical aspects amenable only to the intervention of the expert. Disability is located here in the impaired body of the individual where limbs and organs do not function in accordance with 'normal' expectations. It is those malfunctioning limbs and organs that are the cause of disability. As a consequence of this biological understanding of disability, people with a disability are therefore deemed to be dependent on the expertise of the medical profession in order to either 'cure' or minimize their problems. Such an approach requires the fitting of prosthetics, for instance, or perhaps certain forms of 'corrective' surgery. In this model, a person with a disability is held to be a passive social actor, who is either incapable or not expert enough to make decisions concerning how they lead their lives and is denied access to the decision-making processes that may govern their medical or social care.

In the social model, disability is located not in the body of the individual person but in society where negative attitudes, barriers and cultural prejudices in relation to disabled people's bodies are the source of disability. There are many examples of prejudicial images and stereotypes of disability in society and in popular culture. For example, in many traditional European fairy tales (in particular the Brothers Grimm's original version) the wicked or evil character is often connoted by physical difference. The use of physical difference to indicate evil is notable in the tale of *Rumplestiltskin*, for example, where the eponymous villain is depicted as a 'deformed' and physically different being. The association of bodily difference and evil is also evident in Shakespeare. The troubled King Richard III in the play of that name has a 'humpback'. The sign of physical difference is used once again to indicate the outsider or evil; in the case of this play, that the king is of questionable character. In contemporary culture, such stereotyping still persists. In the various Austin Powers films, for example, the main protagonist, Dr. Evil, is facially scarred and portrayed as being physically different, as are many of the James Bond villains, of which he is a caricature.

Physical barriers are also easy to identify that lead to people with disabilities being excluded from wider society. A great deal of architecture and public and private buildings are still inaccessible for people with disabilities. These barriers include not just the more obvious instances of stairs, which may or may not inhibit people with mobility impairments, but also colour schemes, for example, which create potential difficulties for people with visual impairments in differentiating between doors and walls. Crucially, constructing a built environment that is fully accessible to disabled people does not just benefit that particular group of users, it also benefits a wide range of other users who also can be subject to exclusion. This list includes women with young children or older people, basically anyone who does not accord with the fit, healthy, able-bodied (probably male) user for whom most buildings arguably appear to be designed.

In the social model, the disabled person is a fully active social actor who is central to deciding what occurs in relation to their health and social care. With the disabled person constituted as an active social actor, health professionals are thereby required to interact in a particular way. Partnership becomes the preferred mode of interaction.

Debate has been growing recently, however, concerning the social model. While not abandoning its main tenets of there being a strong social aspect to disability, in terms of the discriminatory attitudes and physical barriers as just outlined, disquiet focuses on the role of the body and the physical aspects of being a disabled person. Tom Shakespeare (2006), for instance, has drawn attention to how the social model can be dismissive of understanding the pain and suffering that can be associated with certain disabilities. Much of these criticisms relate to the history of how the social model of disability was developed by both academics and activists within the disability rights movement (Oliver, 1990; Swain et al., 2003).

Ultimately, these criticisms are not advanced to dispense with the social model of disability. They are put forward to add nuance and subtlety and to open up new areas for conceptual development and further research.

Whatever the outcome of this debate, what is clear is that disability is a very complex concept that requires understanding on a variety of different levels, including the cultural, the social, the psychological and the biological. Difficulties will remain in trying to establish the causes of disability. Is it just society or is there more to it than that? It may, therefore, be useful to describe disability as a common state of being that emerges out of complex social, psychological, intellectual, emotional and biological processes where some form of social difference is attached to people who are deemed or who self-identify as being disabled.

REFERENCES AND FURTHER READING

National Statistics (2006) *Focus on Health*. Basingstoke: Palgrave Macmillan.
Oliver, M. (1990) *The Politics of Disablement*. London: Macmillan.
Shakespeare, T. W. (2006) *Disability Rights and Wrongs*. London: Routledge.
Swain, J., French, S. and Cameron, C. (2003) *Controversial Issues in a Disabling Society*. Milton Keynes: Open University Press.
WHO (World Health Organization) (2004) *The Global Burden of Disease: 2004 Update*. Geneva: World Health Organization.

C. Y.

Alternative or complementary medicine

Alternative medicine embraces any medical practice that falls outside the boundaries of conventional western medicine. Some commentators use the term 'complementary medicine' to imply that non-conventional medicine can be used in conjunction with western biomedicine rather than as a radical alternative.

Trying to be more specific about what exactly constitutes alternative or complementary therapy and to advance a precise definition is more problematic, however. Why the difficulty arises relates to the sheer number and diversity of alternative therapies that are currently on offer in contemporary society. A large variety of quite different practices and therapies can be recognized as being alternative or complementary therapies. These include shiatsu massage, angel therapy, homeopathy acupuncture and kinesiology, to identify just a few. What each therapy offers and involves is also highly varied. Even though all alternative or complementary therapies profess some form of holistic approach (an important point that is expanded upon later), they are often highly different in emphasis and in their practice. As West (1993) notes, the emphasis can be physical, psychological or spiritual. For example, shiatsu is a form of therapeutic massage that relies on the physical manipulation of the body, while angel therapy relies on contacting supernatural entities for guidance and healing.

West also identifies other differences. Some alternative or complementary therapies require a trained practitioner, who has undertaken what can be extensive training, requiring attendance on courses and passing rigorous exams. Such formality is in line with what Saks (2003) has identified as an increasing trend towards professionalization within alternative and complementary medicine. Others can be on a 'do-it-yourself' basis, where individuals gain some level of knowledge from sources such as manuals or websites, while other therapies yet lie between those two poles, with people self-appointing themselves as healers after reading a few books, for example. There is also one further distinction as suggested by Saks (1992) and it is to be found in the subtle but yet important difference between what is termed 'alternative' and what is termed 'complementary'. Those practices that subscribe to the 'alternative' option often emphasize a rejection of or contrast to mainstream biomedicine and seek to distance themselves from it, while those that are termed 'complementary' wish to be regarded as being allied to mainstream medicine but offering a different approach that seeks to augment rather than fully challenge biomedicine.

The actual efficacy (whether the various practices work) of alternative or complementary medicine is not the concern of this entry. That judgement remains the subject of a very heated and passionate debate that currently indicates no sign of abating or even being satisfactorily resolved. It is more fruitful to instead explore why at this point in time so many people in western societies are turning to other approaches that look either to other cultures or back in time in order to maintain or improve their general health and well-being or to overcome illness. This shift in people's preferences is especially interesting given that contemporary western societies emerged out of the Enlightenment project of scientific truth and rationality.

The reasons are many, sometimes contradictory, but ultimately are related to wider developments in society. Listed below are reasons why alternative and complementary therapies are becoming increasingly popular:

Holism is an important element of all alternative or complementary therapies. The emphasis here is on the person in their totality, seeking a unified understanding of mind and body, through contextualizing an individual's experiences and circumstances. The integrated approach found in the alternative and complementary therapies stands in stark contrast to mainstream medicine that usually offers an atomized approach. The physical body rather than the person is the focus of intervention in mainstream medicine. It is in encounters between practitioners and clients that this difference in orientation is perhaps most visible. The standard time a western physician or doctor spends with a client can be a matter of minutes due to a variety of pressures and influences often beyond their control. The thrust of the encounter is identifying as quickly as possible the cause of an illness. In doing so, the wider aspects of someone's life can be ignored. Encounters with alternative practitioners can conversely be up to an hour; the focus is on the person as a whole with maximum time centred on that person.

The influence of consumer culture also exerts an influence and follows on from the above point. Contemporary society emphasizes the centrality of service, of professionals being there to provide a service as opposed to occupying a position of authority as can be the case in mainstream medicine. For the reasons outlined above, alternative and complementary therapies offer a practitioner–client relationship that parallels the consumerist provider–customer relationship.

Medicalization and increased media coverage of the 'risks' involved with conventional medicine have been other spurs for alternative and complementary therapies. Alternative and complementary therapies can appear to be 'safer' and less controlling than conventional approaches.

As mentioned earlier, the debate on the issues of effectiveness and safety carries on unabated, but it is the perceptions of risk and safety that are important. The alternative therapies are perceived to be safer with their connections to nature and images of purity and simplicity. This connection with nature emerges in the next point too.

Older sections of the population still adhere to some of the counter-culture symbolism and beliefs of their youth. The current older generation, or, more precisely, the post-war baby-boomers, were young during the 1960s. At that time, hippie youth subculture prioritized nature and natural symbols, with all things natural being regarded as being of greater value than science and technology against which they were rebelling. Now as a reasonably affluent part of society, this cohort of older people have the financial ability to enact their younger beliefs. Alternative and complementary therapies, which also often invoke natural symbolism, can therefore be of interest and appeal to that group.

Younger doctors who have trained and grown up in a culture where complementary therapies and medicines are more widely accepted in turn may be more inclined than their older peers to see such approaches as being useful and to recommend them to patients and clients.

We are now living in what some sociologists term a post-modernist society that rejects single solution narratives (such as the **biomedical model**) and is more embracing of different discourses and ideologies existing at the same time. This mindset leads to a more 'pick-and-mix' culture where people are happy to simultaneously engage with sometimes apparently contradictory practices and discourses. So, for instance, someone may be receiving health care treatment from the NHS but decide to additionally augment it with a homeopathic cure.

In Western high-income countries, the main causes of premature death are the chronic illnesses. As a host of research indicates, chronic illness often tests the limits and abilities of medical science, and also the confidence people have in medical science. Medical procedures and drug therapies may not work or have highly unpleasant side effects. For people with chronic illnesses, alternative and complementary therapies may therefore provide some form of hope after the perceived failings of contemporary medicine.

For all that alternative and complementary medicines and therapies appear to pose a radical challenge to biomedicine, elements of alternative and complementary therapies do not always accord with the social model either. A strong individualism is apparent in many such therapies, where it is the individual who seeks out a cure for their problems. Absent here is the presence of wider and deeper social influences, such as class, ethnicity and gender that are central to the social model's explanation of health and illness.

It will be interesting to observe how debates and criticisms of alternative and complementary medicine and therapies develop and possibly are resolved. One notable development has been a call for 'integrated medicine' where the best of both mainstream and complementary medicines and therapies are combined. Again, there is no 'definitive' proof that such an approach is more effective than conventional medical approaches. Ultimately though, alternative and complementary therapies and medicines suggest two important lessons for studying health. First, rational medical science does not always provide the answers to the questions people have about their health. Decisions and motives concerning health are just as likely, if not more so, to be influenced by wider social developments. Second, the current popularity of alternative and complementary medicine and therapies indicates that biomedicine may not be as powerful and as hegemonic in society as it once was.

See also: *The social model of health; and Risk society.*

REFERENCES AND FURTHER READING

McQuaide, M. (2005) 'The rise of alternative health care: a sociological account', *Social Theory and Health*, 3: 286–301.

Saks, M. (1992) *Alternative Medicine in Britain*. London: Clarendon.

Saks, M. (2003) *Orthodox and Alternative Medicine: Politics, Professionalization and Health Care*. London: Sage.

West, R. (1993) 'Alternative medicine: prospects and speculation', in N. Black, D. Boswell, A. Gray, S. Murphy and J. Popay (eds), *Health and Disease: A Reader*. Milton Keynes: Open University Press.

C. Y.

Quality of life measures

The concept of 'quality of life' can be found in two distinct areas of health and social research. The first has its origins in early twentieth-century eugenics, and was used as a descriptive assessment of presumed life patterns resulting from a chronic condition, in particular, infants with severe disabilities. These assessments combined clinical judgement (including moral and social concerns) with a set of economic rationale in order to establish a systematic case for non-treatment of those whose physical and cognitive abilities differed from the norm (Koch, 2000: 420). The second, more socially-orientated conception of quality of life first emerged in the 1920s and was utilized in order to consider social concerns about the general life or 'social health' of communities and the individuals and groups which constituted the said communities. These concerns became pronounced in the 1970s in North America and Western Europe, as the post-war optimism about the benefits of welfare states and the opportunities offered by technological developments began to be widely questioned. Today, this set of concerns continues apace with social and environmental concerns about the stresses of work on individual health and the consequences of the internal combustion engine and nuclear power. The more recent manifestations of this focus on the quality of life of communities are a concern with *social cohesion* and *social capital* (discussed under **Social inequalities in health**).

Focusing on health-related quality of life (HRQL), the early twentieth-century concern with the assessment of those with physical and cognitive impairments gradually moved away from the dubious ethics of non-treatment towards a quantitative concern to measure functional disability. This was primarily for the purposes of planning, assessing the outcomes of health service provision, and of clinical decision-making generally. These concerns with prospective (future-orientated) assessments of chronic illness and disability in order to effectively manage (some would say ration) health care resources and plan for care have, since the 1980s, led to the development of a series of quantitative 'quality of life' measurement instruments to ascertain the perceived health status of specific population groups (the 'elderly', ethnic minorities, the 'depressed'). However, the direct concern of these instruments is less with ascertaining the social contributors to the life quality than with the evaluation of health outcomes for particular population groups.

The emergence of scales to measure subjective perceptions of health, and therefore to act (initially) as a supplement to clinical diagnosis, began in the mid-twentieth century with the development of measures of psychiatric disorders. These early psychiatric instruments which employed a limited number of items were used to demonstrate that neurosis could be measured relatively easily across large groups. The success of these measurement instruments reflected a unique feature of psychiatric disorders, that the expressed symptoms were themselves the 'pathology' (which would not be the case for the physical symptoms of an organic disease). For example, those who scored highly in terms of levels of anxiety could then be described as having an anxiety disorder, and those who reported being depressed could be labelled as having clinical depression. It was precisely because these psychological symptoms were also 'subjective', that it later became possible to incorporate these types of questions into broader measures of subjective health status. Questions such as 'I have lost interest in my appearance' taken from the 1983 Hospital Anxiety and Depression Scale, could be integrated into subsequent Quality of Life instruments, e.g., 'How satisfied are you with the way your body looks?', found in the World Health Organization Quality of Life (WHOQOL–100) scale (Armstrong et al., 2007).

From the 1980s onwards, there has been an exponential increase in HRQL measurement instruments and associated publications. The large variety and popularity of these instruments reflect the wide range of population groups that are now subject to interrogation about their quality of life (from the elderly to those with mental health problems, to those with cognitive and physical impairments, the socially stressed and others), which in turn determines whether a disease-specific or a generic measurement instrument is to be employed. The limitations of generic scales (such as the SF-36 described below) is that they may not address topics of particular relevance for a given disease or medical intervention. On the other hand, although more disease-orientated measures offer greater specificity, this is often achieved at the expense of generalizability. The variety of instruments also reflects the contested nature of quality of life and the range of theoretical assumptions concerning the dimensions of HRQL, and the proxies for quality of life which are chosen for translation into measurement items. The range of theoretical assumptions concerning the nature of quality of life that can be found most frequently in measurement scales includes the following (Bowling, 2005):

- classic models of quality of life rooted in notions of subjective well-being and/or happiness;
- needs-based approaches derived from Maslow's hierarchy of human needs;
- models which emphasize social-psychological constructs such as self-efficacy, perceived behavioural control and personal autonomy;
- social expectations approaches based on the perceived gap between desired and actual life circumstances;
- a phenomenological understanding of quality of life which conceives it as dependent upon individual value systems rather than upon a set of universal conceptualizations;
- one of the most frequently found assumptions concerning the measurement of quality of life is that it can be defined in functional terms, usually in relation to physicality but sometimes also in terms of social functioning (discussed in more detail under **Functionality**).

MEASUREMENT ISSUES

Descriptions of health are typically placed on a nominal, ordinal or an interval scale. A *nominal* scale uses numbers to classify a characteristic or item. This type of scale is often used as means for the comparative evaluation of an intervention (before and after). The *ordinal* scale is used where objects in one category of the scale are to be ranked against each other in some way, for example, 'how does X compare with Y?'. The *interval* scale is characterized by a common and constant unit of measurement such as temperature, and is a precise quantitative scale; measures of health status and disability because of their subjective qualities rarely reach an interval-level of measurement. As Bowling (2005) has noted, problems associated with the validity of measuring health outcomes (does an indicator measure the object that it purports to?) using such measurement scales are rife. This is because no 'gold standard' of health exists against which the indices of health status used in a particular scale can be compared; health is an essentially a subjective state.

EXAMPLE OF AN HRQL INSTRUMENT

The Short Form (SF)-36: This is the most commonly used measurement of generic health status (its popularity reflecting its brevity and coverage), and as such its findings dominate the quality of life literature. This 36-item questionnaire was developed in the USA in the early 1990s, and can be administered by oneself, an interviewer, on the telephone or on the computer – it takes about five minutes to complete. The instrument measures eight dimensions of health status: physical functioning (10 items), social functioning (2 items), role limitations due to physical problems (4 items), role limitations due to emotional problems (3 items), mental health (5 items), energy/vitality (4 items), pain (2 items), general health perception (5 items), and one item about the individual's perceptions of changes in their health over the past year. The instrument claims to measure positive and not just negative assessments of individual health status. In the original scoring method, the item scores for each of the eight dimensions are summed and translated using a scoring algorithm, into a scale from 0 (poor health) to 100 (good health). The validity of the SF-36 can be judged by the fact that it is the most widely evaluated generic health status instrument used across the world. In particular, it has been reported that it is more sensitive to graduations in poor health than other broad health instruments. It has good validity in a number of clinical areas associated with physical morbidities, and also is of value in screening for psychiatric disorders, particularly depression. In terms of its reliability, high inter-item co-efficiency correlations have been reported for its sub-scales. The health perception dimension in particular has good correlation with the energy/fatigue scale, although less well with the pain scale.

Finally, one of the interesting features of research that has examined how lay people define their own quality of life (in contrast to the constructed HRQL measurement instruments) is its multi-dimensionality, embracing a positive psychological outlook, emotional well-being (which includes good relationships with family and friends), physical health, personal safety, access to good services, not being dependent upon others, and of course sufficient money (Bowling, 1995). This is in clear contrast to the use of unidimensional indicators (psychological well-being; functionality; social support, happiness, etc.) of quality of life traditionally found in both the broad generic and disease-specific measurement scales described above, whatever might be said about the range of independent or causal variables included in its formulation.

REFERENCES AND FURTHER READING

Armstrong, D., Lilford, R., Ogden, J. and Wessely, S. (2007) 'Health-related quality of life and the transformation of symptoms', *Sociology of Health and Illness*, 29: 570–83.

Bowling, A. (1995) 'What things are important in people's lives? A survey of the public's judgements to inform scales of health related quality of life', *Social Science and Medicine*, 10: 1447–62.

Bowling, A. (2005) *Measuring Health: A Review of Quality of Life Measurement Scales*, 3rd edn, Maidenhead: Open University Press.

Koch, T. (2000) 'Life quality vs the "quality of life": assumptions underlying prospective quality of life instruments in health care planning', *Social Science and Medicine* 51: 419–27.

I. C.

Functionality

Functionality as a measure of health would appear to be more straight-forward to assess than health-related quality of life (HRQL) (see **Quality of life measures**), but this is not necessarily the case. The range of social contexts and the existence of culture differences represent and are reflected in different challenges presented to the human body, and this in turn affects the ways in which health functionality can be and is assessed.

One widely used measure of functionality seeks to assess the performance of an individual in relation to what are termed 'activities of daily living' (ADLs). ADLs are essentially a list of everyday activities which involve both physical capacities (walking, holding, seeing, hearing, mobility, climbing stairs, etc.) and social capacities (cooking, driving, managing finances, etc.). This conceptualization is utilized within the field of health and social care in order to assess the functionality of those living with a physical impairment or limiting chronic illness. The application of ADLs in this context reflects the influence of the World Health Organization's (WHO) 1980 international classification system which assessed the impact of disease on 'social functioning' in terms of following a path from 'impairment' to 'disability', and then onto 'handicap' (WHO, 1980). In 1998, the WHO revised this classification so that 'functioning' became an umbrella term for all body functions, activities and participation, while 'disability' became the general term utilized for impairments, activity limitation or restrictions (WHO, 1998). The revised classification thus drew a clear distinction between 'functioning' and general health status. Functioning in the context of the WHO definition is directly related to the ability to perform one's roles and participate in life, which the social consequences of living with a disability may limit or prevent. Functional status is therefore only one component of health, and is primarily concerned with assessing the effects of disease (Bowling, 2005: 4).

Implicit in the use of ADL-type measures of health is a set of shared social expectations and values. In developed societies these would be typically concerned with whether an individual can manage to live by themselves in their own home without support, be able to drive a car, access and use the internet, etc. By way of contrast, in less-developed societies, functionality (if assessed at all) may mean the ability to walk several miles to access services, draw water and light a fire. Clearly these functional demands change over time as societies themselves change and develop. Functionality, then, in the context of activities of daily living, is not a fixed and universal set of social requirements.

This leads onto a consideration of the understanding of functionality in the sociology of health literature where a wide range of studies can be found that have explored the understandings of both individuals and a variety of social groups of the constituents of 'health'. Blaxter (1990) in her summary of a large national 'Health and Lifestyle' survey derived (not pre-selected) a number of broad categories from the survey respondents' own statements of what they perceived to be the constituents of 'health'. A range of perspectives were found in the survey, but 'health' defined as the ability to effectively function socially recurred most often, particularly among the elderly and the working class. In an earlier study of socially disadvantaged families in Scotland, Blaxter and Paterson (1982) found that the majority of the mothers and daughters who were interviewed defined their health in this functional way. That is, in terms of their ability to carry on normal everyday roles and meet associated social expectations. The phrase, 'never having a day's illness' was found to be used as a (positive) moral characteristic of individuals, although it certainly did not mean that these same people never had a diagnosable illness. These authors found little evidence of a positive concept of health, and it was concluded that these functional conceptions of health were clearly influenced by the experience of a high prevalence of ill-health in the working-class community being studied. Jocelyn Cornwall (1984), in her study of a working-class community in Bethnal Green in East London, similarly found the way people thought about their health in terms of a 'cheerful stoicism' evident in the refusal of those women whom she interviewed to worry or complain or to be morbid. These accounts also demonstrate the possibilities of 'normal' illness. This perspective (as well as a disdainful view of the stoicism of men!) is reflected in the following interview excerpt drawn from the study:

> Most men are babyish, aren't they? They couldn't stand the pain. Especially labour pain, they'd never survive … I'd say that women have more aches and pains than men, but, as I say, when you've got a family, you'll find a woman will work till she's dropping.

This finding that the working class in particular perceive the healthy body as primarily a 'means to an end' or even as a 'machine' (which may require servicing from medical professionals in order to run efficiently) is also found in the work of Pierre Bourdieu (1977). Bourdieu's anthropological work within France concluded that the working class tended to have an instrumental understanding of their health (the notion of the body as physical capital). By way of contrast, the middle classes/professions were seen to perceive their health in a very different way, as a 'personal project'. Health was perceived as being under their own personal control, and as reflecting the outcome of particular 'lifestyle' choices. This approach reinforces the idea that the notion of 'health' is very much a social and cultural construction reflecting the realities of life for different social groups.

The notion of health as related to social functionality also underpins Zola's (1973) 'help-seeking' model (see **Models of health behaviour**) which concluded that the lay public do not seek the help of health professionals or access the formal health care system immediately they perceive physical symptoms. People were typically found to initially try and find ways to accommodate to their symptoms, that is, until they impinge upon, or prevent 'normal role' functioning. It was only at this point of 'crisis' that help would be sought from health care professionals.

Finally, it should also be pointed out in relation to the notion of functionality in the context of health that clinicians frequently utilize the term 'function' to denote the normal operation of discrete body systems. This is a mechanistic and reductionist use of the term, and has no connection to the holistic sense of social functioning.

functionality

REFERENCES

Blaxter, M. (1990) *Health and Lifestyles*. London: Tavistock/Routledge.

Blaxter, M. and Paterson, S. (1982) *Mothers and Daughters: A Three-generation Study of Health, Attitudes and Behaviour*. London: Heinemann Educational.

Bourdieu, P. (1977) *Outline of a Theory of Practice*. Cambridge: Cambridge University Press.

Bowling, A. (2005) *Measuring Health: A Review of Quality of Life Measurement Scales*, 3rd edn. Maidenhead: Open University Press.

Cornwall, J. (1984) *Hard-earned Lives*. London: Tavistock.

WHO (World Health Organization) (1980) *International Classification of Impairments, Disabilities and Handicaps*. Geneva: WHO.

WHO (World Health Organization) (1998) *International Classification of Impairments, Activities and Participation: A Manual of Dimensions of Disablement and Functioning*. Geneva: WHO.

Zola, I. (1973) 'Pathways to the Doctor: from person to patient', *Social Science and Medicine*, 7: 677–89.

I. C.

key concepts in
health studies

Part 2
The Human
Life Course

The life course

The concepts of 'lifespan' and 'lifecycle' are can be found within medical and social gerontological texts in reference to the process of ageing (from birth to death). The application of these overarching terms does have its difficulties because they suggest a predictable and universal series of biological stages through which all people must inevitably pass. In practice, while birth, maturation and death are constants of the human condition, they set only the most general limitations on individual and group experiences.

The 'life course' concept is now widely utilized within Health and Social Studies of ageing because it frames these biological process in a much more dynamic way. Individual biological development is seen to take place within a social context. This approach 'enables variations and continuities in the social status that individuals experience as they mature to be emphasised' (Hockey and James, 1993). Such life course patterns constitute the sequence of participation in various life domains that span from birth to death. That is, from the beginnings of early full-time education through the school years and the sequences of education and training activities, followed by entry into the labour market, employment careers, and interruptions of labour force participation, for example, to have children, then retirement to end of life. Traditional life course patterns would include the years growing up in families, leaving parental homes, partnership formation, marriages and parenthood; and regional mobility (see Hepworth, 2000, for further examples).

The life course approach emphasizes the dynamics of social roles played by individuals over time. Here, the connected concepts of *trajectories* (sometimes conceived as *stages*) and *transitions* are drawn upon in order to contextualize the ways in which these social roles change and develop over an extended period of time. *Trajectories* reflect the changing level of individual participation within social structures, for example, schooling, work, marriage and parenthood. While *transitions* mark the beginning and end of trajectories and give them their particular form and meaning; examples would include the transition from child to adult, and from regular employment to retirement. Transitions are therefore typically of shorter duration than trajectories. In practice, the dynamics of the life course are characterized by the interlocking of multiple role trajectories for individuals, reflecting their participation in a range of roles at the levels of social interaction, organizations, and subsystems of the society (MacMillan and Copher, 2005: 859).

The life course is therefore socially and culturally constructed, and experienced and understood in different ways by different groups of people in different historical times and geographical places:

> There is a social dimension to human life which cannot be reduced to a set of bodily imperatives. Thus 'ageing' is not simply a matter of organic maturation and decay, for the way in which these processes are understood and their import for societies' members differ cross-culturally. (Hockey and James, 1993: 23)

Historical and cultural changes within Britain in the past few decades have brought about significant shifts in the 'transitions' of the life course for many. Indeed, it is now frequently stated that we are witnessing the decline in the significance of biological age and the accompanying loosening of age timetables for many adult transitions. The early adult years are a good case in point, where just decades ago, leaving home, completing schooling, finding employment, getting married, and having children all occurred in a predictable and socially required series of steps, and over a relatively short period of time. Entry into adulthood now takes longer and happens in more individualized ways. Some of these experiences, such as getting married and having children as soon as possible, are becoming decoupled from each other; the 'transition' to parenthood not occurring for increasing numbers of people until they are in their 30s. Indeed, it is now not uncommon to find an increasing number of women making a positive choice not to have children in favour of a career or other personal reasons. Some of these steps in early adulthood also now happen in different orders or with different spacing (Settersten, 2009). The norm in the 1950s, for example, was for people to get married in their early 20s, yet by the 1980s this was occurring later in life, frequently after a period of cohabitation.

Research in the field of health inequalities (see **Social inequalities in health**) increasingly utilizes a life course approach to the understanding of the important role of early life factors in later adult mortality and morbidity; inequalities in health as experienced over the entire life course not in its latter stages. Contemporary studies based on longitudinal data for individuals using a life course approach repeatedly show the importance of early-life factors for overall mortality at older ages, as well as for mortality in specified diseases (Kuh and Ben-Shlomo, 2004). While epidemiological studies based on population totals do provide a large overview of health inequalities across the age range, life course studies conducted at the individual level give specificity and make it possible to test causal models. Life course models using longitudinal individual-level data (for example, the work of Palloni et al., 2009, which draws on the 1958 British birth cohort longitudinal data) for analyzing adult mortality include such factors as mother's condition during the foetal stage, birth weight, height, prevalence of diseases, and sometimes information from blood tests (Bengsston and Mineau, 2009). The life course approach thus conceives life and health chances as being constituted as much by social context as biological development. Social advantages and disadvantages in relation to individual health outcomes are seen to cluster cross-sectionally (in relation to an individual's socio-economic class position) and accumulate longitudinally (their relative exposure to health hazards over the course of a lifetime) (Blane et al., 1997).

The life course concept is able to draw attention to the importance of role change over time (trajectories and transitions) in order to link early life social and health experiences to those of later life for individuals. This focus on the ageing process as reflecting role changes over time can be further developed by thinking in terms of two interrelated but analytically separable aspects of change over time – 'biographical' and 'historical' (Bury, 2000). *Biographical time* refers to the processes, experiences and events that occur during an individual's lifetime. While some of these experiential aspects are highly individual, other aspects are influenced by the social context within which that person lives, and by age-related structures that influence biographical experiences, i.e., school leaving, retirement. *Historical time*, on the other hand, points to the importance of age *cohort effects*. This approach is able to conceive the life course of individuals in the context of the experiences of particular and unique generational groups who age in specific historical circumstances. For example, the impact of experiencing early life without automatic access to free and universal health services, as is the case for those born before the inception of the welfare state, on the long-term health of this particular cohort.

the life course

REFERENCES AND FURTHER READING

Bengsston, T. and Mineau, G. (2009) 'Early-life effects on socio-economic performance and mortality in later life: a full life-course approach using contemporary and historical sources', *Social Science and Medicine*, 68(9): 1561–4.

Blane, D., Bartley, M. and Davey Smith, G. (1997) 'Disease aetiology and materialist explanations of socioeconomic mortality differentials', *European Journal of Public Health*, 7: 385–91.

Bury, M. (2000) 'Health, ageing and the lifecourse', in S. Williams, J. Gabe and M. Calnan, (eds), *Health, Medicine and Society*. London: Routledge, pp. 87–106.

Hepworth, M. (2000) *Stories of Ageing*. Maidenhead: Open University Press.

Hockey, J. and James, A. (1993) *Growing Up and Growing Old: Ageing and Society*. London: Sage.

Hockey, J. and James, A. (2003) *Social Identities across the Life Course*. London: Palgrave.

Kuh, D. and Ben-Shlomo, Y. (eds) (2004) *A Life Course Approach to Chronic Disease Epidemiology*, 2nd edn. Oxford: Oxford University Press.

MacMillan, R. and Copher, R. (2005) 'Families in the life course: interdependency of roles, role configurations, and pathways', *Journal of Family and Marriage*, 67: 858–79.

Palloni, A., Milesi, C., White, R. G. and Turner, A. (2009) 'Early childhood health, reproduction of economic inequalities, and the persistence of health and mortality differentials', *Social Science and Medicine*, 68(9): 1574–82.

Settersten, R. (2009) 'It takes two to tango: the (un)easy dance between life-course sociology and life-span psychology', *Advances in Life Course Research*, 14(1–2): 74-81.

I. C.

Childbirth

Childbirth outwardly appears to be a 'natural' biological process. Yet, as with so much else discussed in this book, childbirth has as much – if not more – to do with society and culture as it does with biology. This more holistic approach is central to a Health Studies understanding of childbirth, where the medical and biological elements of childbirth are but elements of a much wider and deeper perspective. The cultural differences in childbirth and the medicalization of childbirth are two key aspects of a more rounded approach to understanding childbirth and fall under particular consideration here. Doing so highlights the extent to which social processes and social constructions frame and influence the act and experience of childbirth, while also identifying tensions between 'natural' and 'artificial' approaches to the act of childbirth.

Comparing different societies can provide useful insights into how childbirth and the experience of being pregnant are framed and bound up in cultural norms and practices. Even between countries that one would expect to be fairly similar in culture, and therefore similar in how childbirth is socially constructed, notable and interesting differences occur. Comparing childbirth in the Netherlands and the United Kingdom provides such a contrast. Despite both being European, capitalist nations, the cultural role and significance of childbirth are quite different in each country (Van Teijlingen 2000). In the Netherlands childbirth is regarded as being a 'natural' and healthy state for a woman. Contact with the medical profession is restricted to as few encounters as possible, and mainly at the outset of the pregnancy. Once it is established that all is well with both mother and baby, the main health professional involved in caring for and supporting the pregnant woman is a midwife. Delivery takes place at home, with the state providing home support for a short period after the birth. This understanding of childbirth is quite different from that experienced in the UK. Childbirth is perceived not so much as a natural healthy state but as a state of medical and biological risk. Consequently, the women experiences her pregnancy as a medical state under the surveillance (if not control) of doctors and obstetricians. Medical examinations are routine, with the birth located in a hospital. The Netherlands, notably, has a slightly better record in babies surviving birth than in the UK.

The experience of childbirth in the UK as outlined above is an example of **medicalization**, the process whereby a phenomena or situation that was formerly considered to be 'natural' is subsumed into the biomedical sphere. Much of the sociological and feminist scholarship on childbirth has focused on this process of medicalization, and in particular the ways in which control over childbirth has been removed from women and been replaced by patriarchal medical power. Medicalization reorders and changes women's experiences of maternity so that it becomes akin to the experience of being ill. The dominance of medicalization is reflected in the increasing numbers of babies born in hospital, the associated presence of medical technology, as well as the continual biomedical surveillance of the mother. How this situation came about and the implications for women are expanded upon below.

Historically, the medical profession (the emergent speciality of Obstetrics and Gynaecology) succeeded in displacing midwifes as the occupation who could claim to have the appropriate expertise to manage childbirth. The title 'midwife' was derived from the old Anglo-Saxon *mit wif* (literally meaning 'with the woman'), and for much of history, care of the pregnant woman and assisting in the delivery of the baby were in the female domain and outside the control of both men and the incipient medical profession. The arrival of biomedicine in the eighteenth century marked a fundamental shift in who oversaw childbirth and where child-birth was to take place. The emerging medical profession sought to deni-grate rivals that potentially prevented the medical profession achieving total and hegemonic control over health and healing and increasingly side-lined women and the midwife. The actual process unfolded over time and it was not until the founding of obstetrics in the 1830s that the (male) medical professions succeeded in claiming this part of life as their own. As has been noted, the process of male obstetricians taking over from female midwives often involved invoking spurious claims concerning the validity and efficacy of their approach (Oakley, 1976), in addition to the advan-tages afforded to male obstetricians by often coming from a higher social class than the female midwives.

The medicalization of childbirth represents a loss of control for mothers, with each of the stages of labour being guided not by the woman responding to her innate understandings of her requirements but prompted by medical technology. Martin (2003) has also suggested that control over childbirth by the medical profession is not only real-ized through the use of technology in hospital settings. She argues that women have internalized patriarchal (male power) ideologies, which, in turn, make women act in a compliant attitude towards the male obstetricians. A clash of perspectives between the woman in labour and the medical profession can also occur. For the women, the experi-ence of giving birth is an element in a wider personal and familial narrative. This holistic focus is in contrast with the obstetrician's perspec-tive of prioritizing the health of the baby above all else. Though, as with other experiences, class and ethnicity also exert an influence. Middle-class women typically can exert more control over childbirth than working-class women.

There has, as Annandale (2009) notes, been concern about the child-birth and medicalization thesis and the notion inherent in critiques of medicalization that 'natural' births are liberating for women, allowing them to reassert control over their labour. As Macintyre (1977) cau-tions, a strong scepticism of a golden age of childbirth ever existing is necessary (see **The life course**). Childbirth in pre-modern times was dangerous and frequently could result in death for both mother and child. Moves to develop a 'midwifery model' or feminist model of child-birth may, therefore, be seen as a (valid) reaction against the historically

key concepts in
health studies

more recent trend of the medicalization of childbirth as opposed to the continuation of a 'pure' tradition that stretches seamlessly back in time. Childbirth has always occurred in and been medicated by social context. What that context is changes over time, of course, and emerges out of the various political and social trends and discourses of a particular time. It may therefore be quite difficult to advance a pure 'natural' model of childbirth. Just because a procedure is constructed as being 'natural' does not entail that it is free of the trappings of medical model approaches to childbirth. As Lupton (2006) has noted, a shift towards 'natural' childbirth does not necessarily break the monopoly of medical professional control. The medical profession can absorb and appropriate this new discourse and exert control there too. Perhaps, at the end of the day, as Brubaker and Dillaway (2008) have suggested, most women may prefer a birth that falls between the two poles of 'medical' and 'natural'.

REFERENCES AND FURTHER READING

Annandale, E. (2009) *Women's Health and Social Change*. London: Routledge.
Brubacker, S. J. and Dillaway, H. (2008) 'Re-examining the meanings of childbirth: Beyond gender and the "natural" v. "medical" dichotomy', in M. Texler Segal and V. Demos (eds), *Advancing Gender Research from the Nineteenth to the Twenty-First Centuries: Advances in Gender Research*, Vol. 12.
Lupton, D. (2006) *Medicine as Culture*. London: Sage.
Macintyre, S. (1977) 'Childbirth: the myth of the Golden Age', *World Medicine*, 12(18): 17–22.
Martin, K. (2003) 'Giving birth like a girl', *Gender and Society*, 17(1): 54–72.
Oakley, A. (1976) 'Wisewoman and medicineman: changes in the management of childbirth', in J. Mitchell and A. Oakley (eds), *The Rights and Wrongs of Women*. London: Penguin.
Van Teijlingen, E. (2000) 'Maternity home care assistants in the Netherlands', in E. van Teijlingen, G. Lewis, P. McCaffery and M. Porter (eds), *Midwifery and the Medicalization of Childbirth*. New York: Nova Science.

C. Y.

childbirth

Childhood

Childhood may seem a fairly unambiguous, or straight-forward and simple enough, concept to be discussing. Childhood for many people simply refers to a period in our lives (usually between 5 to 14 years), which is infused with images of innocence and naivety. In addition to these emotional associations, childhood can also be seen as a time of risk and danger, where fragile bodies can come to harm falling off bicycles or tripping in playgrounds and where that innocence and naivety can lead to dangerous and unsafe encounters with deviant members of the adult world.

On closer inspection, the perspective on childhood outlined above does not strictly hold true. Indeed, much of what is sketched out above only really understands childhood at one particular point in time and in one particular culture. Childhood, or rather a western understanding of childhood as summarized above, is a socially constructed phase both at a particular historical point in a society and in the life course of individuals. Socially constructed here refers to how what may be held or regarded as being 'natural' or 'commonsense' is actually the outcome of particular historical, cultural and social processes. What therefore appears to be a fixed and a stable aspect of daily life and experience is in effect potentially fleeting and contingent. Furthermore, it is also liable to be changed and reordered into some other state of affairs at a future point in time. It may, therefore, be more accurate, as is discussed further in this entry, to refer not to 'childhood' as a singular heterogeneous entity but rather 'childhoods', thereby acknowledging the multiplicity of different ways that childhood is constructed and experienced in different places and at different historical times (Punch, 2003).

Philippe Ariès, a French social historian, has explored the socially constructed basis of childhood in depth. He identifies in his widely read (1962) book *Centuries of Childhood* that during the Middle Ages, for instance, at the age of seven, young people were considered to be adults. As a consequence young people of that time were apprenticed to work on the fields or in some other craft. They were, in effect, not children but young adults and perceived by contemporary society of being both capable of the social duties and of engaging in the responsibilities

key concepts in
health studies

40

associated with adulthood. It was not until the fifteenth century that notions of a separate childhood begin to emerge, though significantly only among the upper classes. This development was mainly in response to religious doctrine concerning children within medieval Christianity. The prevailing discourse at the time was that God perceived children as special beings. It was the advent of industrialization in the modern period and the various ways in which the family became internally differentiated and externally separated from other social domains that laid down the basis of what is taken as childhood today in contemporary western cultures. Critics such as Linda Pollock (1983) have, however, criticized Ariès on a number of grounds relating to his method (analysing artworks mainly) and other aspects of his thesis, particularly in relation to the historical emergence of childhood. Pollock, for instance, has claimed that childhood has always existed to some extent and a continuity exists in how adults and children have related to each other. Despite these criticisms, the central message of Ariès, that childhood is open to some form of social construction, provides a useful insight into understanding and conceptualizing childhood.

By claiming that childhood is open to social construction, one has to be careful, however, not to draw the following inferences. First, just because some element of our lives is socially constructed does not automatically entail that we do not hold deep and 'real' emotional attachments to it. Childhood is a special time in most people's life, whether their own childhood or the childhood of their own offspring. Second, by claiming that childhood is socially constructed, it should not be read as implying that there is not a phase in the biological growth and development of an embodied individual where they possess a body and a mind that is developing toward an adult body and mind. Rather, it is the way in which a society depicts, values and attaches certain symbols to the human body through the life course that is important. Young bodies and young people (or children, in other words) will always continue to exist. It is that not all societies through time would recognize such young people as being 'children', in the manner that certain western societies do so today.

Examining the history of childhood in Britain, for instance, can provide a useful example of how what is perceived and constructed as childhood changes over time. For much of British history, childhood was not seen as a special phase in people's lives. Rather, as soon as a child reached the age when they could engage in productive work, whether in the home or in a workplace such as a factory or mine, they would be expected to do so. In the new mill industries of the Industrial Revolution during the eighteenth century children as young as nine were routinely employed to pick trapped fibres out of fast-moving and dangerous cotton-spinning machines. Often this form of labour led to horrendous accidents with injury or amputation of fingers and hands being common.

This type of childhood work is largely historical in Britain and other western countries today, but in other parts of the world, it remains a feature of everyday life for many children. According to UNICEF (2009), in the world today, one in six children between the ages of five and 14 is involved in child labour, or, put into bald figures, about 158 million children worldwide. Such work is frequently in dangerous unregulated workplaces operating unsafe machinery or working with hazardous chemicals, putting their health at risk. For many child workers, being compelled to work interferes or denies them outright the education that would help to raise both their own and their communities' standard of living in the present and in the future. For the majority of children around the globe, limiting illness and premature death are constant risks. The World Health Organization (WHO, 2007) estimates that nearly 10 million children under the age of five die each year. This works out as over 1000 deaths every hour of every day. The WHO points out that most of these lives could be saved with simple low-cost interventions, such as provision of clean water, adequate labour laws and the provision of schooling.

In western, or high-income nations, childhood is framed by different and perhaps contradictory perceptions of risk and health. One popular construction of childhood is that childhood is in itself a time of high risk, where all children are at risk from accidents, sexual predation or illness. Indeed, childhood and children's health in the West can be characterized as a time of risk management, where all risks, including spills in the playground and 'unhealthy' eating, are the subject of risk management by parents and other adults. Furedi (2002) has criticized this almost hegemonic perception of children being constantly at risk, the downside of which could result in children being too cosseted and overprotected. The possible consequences of this are that children may never gain the skills to deal with risk themselves.

Overall, defining the concept of childhood is not at all straightforward. What is commonly perceived as being childhood is not a universal constant that transcends time and space, but rather is a construction that belongs to a particular culture at a particular point in time. Different ideas of what childhood is and how children should be treated exist across the globe. It is therefore more realistic to refer to 'childhoods', thus accepting the multiple ways of being a 'child' as opposed to maintaining a more simple and inflexible understanding.

See also: *The life course.*

REFERENCES AND FURTHER READING

Ariès, P. (1962) *Centuries of Childhood: A Social History of Family Life*. New York: Alfred, A. Knopf.

Furedi, F. (2002) *Paranoid Parenting: Why Ignoring the Experts May be Best for Your Child*. Atlanta, GA: A Cappella Books.

Mayall, B. (1996) *Children, Health and the Social Order*. Buckingham: Open University Press.

Pollock, L. A. (1983) *Forgotten Children: Parent–child relations from 1500 to 1900*. Cambridge: Cambridge University Press.

Punch, S. (2003) 'Childhoods in the majority world: miniature adults or tribal children?' *Sociology*, 37(2): 277–95.

UNICEF (2009) 'Child protection from violence, exploitation and abuse', 6 March. Available at: http://www.unicef.org/protection/index_childlabour.htm (accessed 17 July 2009).

WHO (World Health Organization) (2007) '10 facts on child health', 29 October. Available at: http://www.who.int/features/factfiles/child_health2/en/index.html (accessed 17 July 2009).

C. Y.

childhood

Family and individual well-being

The relationship between families and health from a life course perspective with its focus on the dynamic, interconnected unfolding *trajectories* and *transitions* (see **The life course**) of individual lives is assessed here. It draws attention to the potential complexity of family role configurations and possible pathways constituted by the interplay of social, economic, and cultural structure with their requirements and proscriptions (MacMillan and Copher, 2005: 861).

In relation to individual health and well-being, the family context of early life can, as Wadsworth (1999) has stated, 'set the trajectory into adulthood'. The processes of individual biological development are strongly mediated by social context, and family circumstances play a key role. The findings of a wide range of social and psychological research have pointed to the strong link between socio-economic position of a family and a child's educational opportunities, which are in turn associated with subsequent occupation and income. Parental concern for and interest in a child's education are also key factors in determining educational attainment and this factor is strongly associated with health-related habits such as smoking, exercise and diet; occupation also being similarly associated with health-related habits (Wadsworth, 1999: 48). The literature on early parenthood, for example, shows a connection with the diminished educational attainment of children, who then have a greater risk of early marriage themselves with a higher potential for divorce, as well as limited possibilities for socio-economic mobility. Parental transitions *out of* marriage (divorce/separation) are also associated with a host of life course 'deficits' in their children, while transitions *into* marriage demonstrate the interlinked lives of spouses, with the consequences of the unfolding life course of one partner having an impact on the other. Thus, the lives of parents and their children as family members are intimately interconnected, with many features of the parents' lives setting the stage for their children's experiences and life chances deep into the life course (evidence cited in MacMillan and Copher, 2005: 862).

Historically, the function of the family and the roles of family members have been significantly influenced by changes in the economic system of production. Before industrialization occurred within Britain, families were

key concepts in health studies

44

not only structures for *reproduction* and the socialization of children, but also units of *production* where all family members worked together to produce their own resources. But with the development of large-scale industrial production, the workplace became separated from the home. These economic developments had the effect of turning virtually all members (it was common for children as young as seven to be working in the mining and cotton manufacturing industry up until the 1840s) of a working family into wage labourers at the beginning of the nineteenth century. Yet by the end of that century paid employment was perceived to be a role limited to adult men because of the improvement in pay and conditions (helping to produce the myth of the single wage family). However, the historical reality was that throughout the twentieth century, the majority of women continued to combine domestic work within the home and outside employment.

The caring role of the family has also experienced dramatic changes in the past hundred years. One explanation has been that this somehow reflects the shift from the 'extended family' (three or more generations of a family living in the same household) taking responsibility for the care of its sick and elderly members, to the 'nuclear family' (consisting of an adult couple united by ties of partnership and parenthood and their socially acknowledged children) of post-war Britain. The nuclear family is seen as having had many of the traditional caring functions of the extended family taken over by the state and its health and social welfare system. This, however, is a simplistic reading of the history of the family. It ignores the fact that the major change in the twentieth century was not a shift towards the nuclear family household group as such, but an absolute decline in the size of families and the greater geographical dispersion of households containing related people. The shift in caring roles is as much about the decline in morbidity and mortality, and the widening employment opportunities for women, as anything to do with the form of the family *per se*. One influential and enduring sociological reading of these changes is that of Young and Wilmott (1961), who argued over 40 years ago that the emotional support provided by family relationships had grown in importance as the family lost some of its material functions; families' roles having become more specialized: 'As the disadvantages of the new industrial and impersonal society have become more pronounced, so the family has become more prized for its power to counteract them'(Young and Wilmott, 1961).

It remains the case within contemporary Britain that it is the family that continues to carry out many of the functions that are so seen to be essential to the reproduction and maintenance of a society. These functions include reproduction, child care, primary socialization, informal health care, economic provision and maintaining the household. It has been argued that these family functions have actually increased in number and become more intensified in recent times.

Contemporary trends in family size and form demonstrate the dynamic shifts that have occurred within family role trajectories. In 2007, for example, 77 per cent of families with dependent children were headed by a married or cohabiting couple. However, there has been a reduction in this type as aproportion of all families over the past 30 years (in 1971, 92 per cent of families were of this type). The percentage of lone mothers rose from seven per cent in 1971 to 22 per cent in 1988, but over the past two decades this proportion has remained more or less the same (see Figure 1). While there has been a continuing increase in divorce, the numbers of second marriages are increasing. There has also been a slow, but often exaggerated, decrease in average family size. The average number of children for all families with dependent children in 1971 was 2.0, while in 2007 it was 1.8. One critical factor in this change is that women are delaying having children until later in life with the percentage of births to women over 30 having doubled in the past 25 years. However, this latter trend is somewhat offset by the very high rate of teenage pregnancies in the UK.

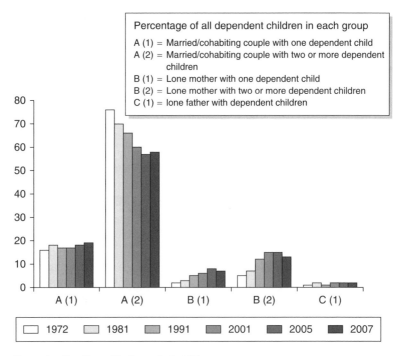

Figure 1   *Families with dependent children*
Source: General Household Survey 2007 (ONS, 2009)

REFERENCES

MacMillan, R. and Copher, R. (2005) 'Families in the life course: interdependency of roles, role configurations, and pathways', *Journal of Marriage and Family*, 67: 858–79.

ONS (Office of National Statistics) (2009) *General Household Survey 2007*. London: Stationery Office.

Wadsworth, M. (1999) 'Early life', in M. Marmot and R. Wilkinson (eds), *Social Determinants of Health*. Oxford: Oxford University Press.

Young, M. and Wilmott, P. (1961) *Family and Kinship in East London*. Harmondsworth: Penguin.

I. C.

Social dependency in older age

A recurring theme in the literature is of old age as a 'social problem'. The elderly population is frequently portrayed by both the government and within the media as an ever-increasing burden on the health and welfare services. Despite the fact that people are today living for longer than ever before and are in better health for longer periods of the life course, older age continues to be viewed problematically. Examples of this understanding include the view that as a society we face a pensions 'problem', a 'long-term care' problem, an 'epidemic' of Alzheimer's disease problem, etc. These ageist attitudes reflect both the way in which older age is socially constructed as a period of social dependency, as well as continuing to shape its structural constitution through state health and social policies.

Dependency in older age can be conceived as some inevitable outcome of biological and physical decline. By way of contrast, the life course approach conceives of individual biological development as taking place within a social context, and identifies a set of social processes as playing an important role in socially structuring dependency in the older members of the population. The 'structured dependency' model derives from the work of both Peter Townsend (1981) and Alan Walker (1981),

social dependency in older age

47

and describes the social process of marginalization that follows a person's exit from the labour market at the point of retirement, both in terms of social isolation, loss of role, and accompanied by severely restricted consumption patterns. These negative consequences of retirement are for many people an outcome of the dependence on the low levels of pension payments that have traditionally existed within the UK, which in turn marks out an association between older age and relative poverty.

A number of constructs flow from, as well as inform the application of structured dependency theory in relation to older age, and these are considered below:

- The consequences of a widening of the *dependency ratio*. This construct is utilized as an expression of the number of 'dependants' such as children and those over retirement age as a ratio of the tax-paying 'working age' population. The ratio has widened in recent years in the majority of developed countries, particularly in Europe. Whether overtly or not, the construct is often deployed to construct the increasing proportion of the population that are elderly as being materially dependent (an 'economic burden') upon the rest of the community (in paid employment).
- The consequences of the increase in life expectancy. In 2004, a woman's life expectancy at birth was 81.0 years compared with 76. 6 years for men (ONS, 2008). This demographic understanding is mobilized to construct the phenomenon of the 'ageing society' in the twenty-first century. This construction assumes that caring by immediate family members is becoming increasingly less common as older people are somehow 'abandoned' by their families to the care of the state, with the outcome being the increasing isolation of the elderly within society (see **Family and individual well-being**). This scenario is conflated by another seemingly inevitable consequence of increased life expectancy, that is, the larger numbers of elderly people living with disability who have become more socially dependent. In practice, what is termed 'healthy life expectancy' defined as the expected years of life in good or fairly good health has increased for all over the past 20 years. In 2004, healthy life expectancy at birth was 68.0 years for men and 70.3 years for women. The amount of time people can then expect to live with a limiting illness or disability has remained more or less constant at around 13 years for men and 16 years for women (ONS, 2008).
- Retirement used as an active policy both by the state and employers to remove elderly people from the workforce when unemployment

is high or when industries require restructuring. That is, exit from the workforce is not based on any medical or health considerations but primarily on industrial and political rationales. This practice is one of the reasons why retirement ages vary so much even among European countries, and why in many of these countries retirement ages have been lowered rather than raised during periods of economic recession. On this basis, the policy of retirement reinforces the construction of older age as a period of dependency.

- The perception of biological ageing (see **Medicalization**) as a problematic pathological process reflects to some degree the development of Geriatrics as an emergent medical specialism in the 1940s. This specialism gradually developed a knowledge base that regarded old age as necessitating specific forms of surveillance through processes of institutionalization, and therapeutic intervention (Armstrong, 1983). It is also contended that this biomedical approach has resulted in a set of *ageist* assumptions concerning the relevance of social inequalities when health outcomes for the older person are considered (see **Social inequalities in health**). Such attitudes lead onto the false assumption (challenged by the life course thesis that emphasizes the accumulation of social advantage and disadvantage and its impact on health outcomes across the entire life course) that the impact of social inequalities upon health somehow moderate in later life as biological age outweighs social factors in influencing health.

- Social dependency in older age perceived as material resource issue. The sociological work of Arber and Ginn (1993) asserts that a key concern of older people is to maintain their independence and autonomy. Greater or lesser access to material and financial resources will be likely to affect a person's chances of achieving relative independence in later life. This situation has relevance for an individual's self-esteem, personal dignity, and well-being in older age. Arber and Ginn's (1993) model is setout in Figure 1 overleaf, and demonstrates the interrelationships of three sets of resources potentially available to older people. These are financial resources (income and wealth), the resource of physical health itself (functional abilities), and the material ability to access to supportive care, both formal and informal – together these form a 'resource triangle'. Access to such resources are conceived of as largely determined by the socioeconomic position an individual held during their period of paid employment in the labour market. However, it is also argued that other social characteristics of the individual such as ethnicity and gender will also influence the likelihood of a person possessing each of the three types of resource. This focus on the importance of material resources in older age is supported by more recent work that has examined the importance of wealth in accessing material resources for good health outcomes in older age. The English Longitudinal Study of Ageing (ELSA) indicates that a strong wealth gradient exists in the greater or lesser likelihood of those reporting poor health among those aged over 50. Those reporting good health in the study had an average (median) wealth around three times higher than that of those reporting fair or poor health; this finding was persistent at all ages (Banks et al., 2003).

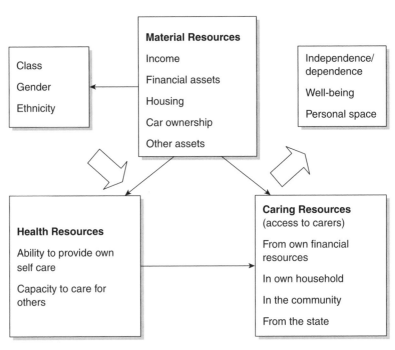

Figure 1   *Three key resources influencing independence and dependence*
Source: Arber and Ginn (1993)

REFERENCES

Arber, S. and Ginn, J. (1993) 'Health and resources in later life', in S. Platt et al. (eds), *Locating Health: Sociological and Historical Explanations.* Aldershot: Avebury Press.

Armstrong, D. (1983) The Political Anatomy of the Body: Medical Knowledge in Britain in the 20th Century, Cambridge: Cambridge University Press.

Banks, J., Karlsen, S. and Oldfield, Z. (2003) 'Socio-economic position', in M. Marmott, J. Banks, and R. Blundell (eds), *Health, Wealth and Lifestyles of the Older Population in England: The 2002 English Longitudinal Study of Ageing*. London: Institute for Fiscal Studies.

ONS (Office of National Statistics) (2008) *Health Expectancy*, available at: www.statistics. gov.uk/cci/nugget.asp?id =934 (accessed May 2009).

Townsend, P. (1981) 'The structured dependency of the elderly', *Ageing and Society*, 1: 5–18.

Walker, A. (1981) 'Towards a political economy of old age', *Ageing and Society*, 1: 73–94.

I. C.

The third age

In contrast to structured dependency theory (see **Social dependency in older age**), the concept of the 'third age' emerged from a quite different social perspective; one that sees the process of ageing in contemporary society as being less constrained by social structural and cultural boundaries than it once was. The widening of consumer society from the 1980s in most western societies was seen by commentators such as Laslett (1989) to have opened up 'lifestyle choices' for the post-retirement individual. This widening of consumerism is seen to have occurred at the same time as the epidemiological phenomenon of the increasing 'disability-free life expectancy' for older people (in which morbidity becomes 'compressed' into just a few years at the very end of life), together with a greater availability of occupational pensions (and therefore less reliance on the minimal state pension in the UK). In combination these factors have enabled commentators such as Gilleard and Higgs (2000: 38–42) to claim that, '[R]etirement is(now) represented as the acquisition of leisure rather than the loss of employment, as people's position in the productive process no longer provides the core of their social and cultural identity.'

The changes that have occurred in the material circumstances and consumption patterns of older people over the past 30 years have enabled some to claim (following Laslett) that older age should be seen not as a single trajectory but rather as encompassing a long 'third age' (50+), before entering the much shorter 'fourth age' of illness and incapacity. Together these processes are seen to have shifted society's perception of the elderly as an identifiable social group marked out by dependency and marginalization. This conceptualisation recognizes the existence of greater social opportunities (and with the associated risks) for older people to take decisions about who they want to be and how they will live their lives after retirement. While pensioner incomes typically decline after retirement, incomes have nevertheless increased over time because of higher lifetime earnings and access to occupational pensions.

> The means by which resources are obtained become less significant than the means by which they are deployed to establish and exemplify a particular lifestyle … [M]any of those recently retired continue or increase their pursuit of consumption-based identities that were not possible for previous generations of retirees. (Gilleard and Higgs, 2000: 32)

The third age perspective therefore challenges the view of the centrality of retirement from work for late-life identity, and posits the experience of older age for many as a golden autumn of consumption and lifestyle opportunities rather than as a period of social dependency. The theoretical assumption being that the consumption of goods and services is now a defining characteristic of social life, having both symbolic as well as practical value (Gilleard et al., 2005), with socio-economic class being a much less culturally significant factor in shaping older people's identities (however what is not in dispute is that socio-economic class continues to act as the key material factor in determining spending patterns).

In the USA, this 'consumptionist' challenge to the traditional stereotypes of older age is also strongly linked with the (largely US) concept of 'successful ageing' (Rowe and Kahn, 1998). Rowe and Kahn defined successful ageing as the absence of disease and disability, the maintenance of cognitive and physical function, and productive social interaction with others. Their main (and essentially politicized) emphasis is that successful ageing is within the control of individuals through the types of lifestyle choices they make and associated health behaviours.

In many respects, the concept of the third age is predicated on individuals having sufficient income and wealth in older age to access the lifestyle choices available through the consumer market. In practice, the average statistical rise in living standards for the over-65s has not been (by definition) experienced equally over the past 20 years. The elderly population is also not a monolithic homogeneous group. The increasing fragmentation of the retired population into those able to enjoy the opportunities that an affluent retirement offers, and those who remain economically and socially dependent on state support, continues in large part to reflect the class-, cohort- and gender-based divisions that exist in wider British society. Alternatively, it is also possible to argue that the structured dependency and third age theories can be reconciled by seeing them as the ideal-type extremes of a spectrum which stretches from dependency to agency in quality of life in early old age (Blane et al., 2004: 2172).

REFERENCES

Blane, D., Higgs, P., Hyde, P. and Wiggins, R. (2004) 'Life course influences on quality of life in early old age', *Social Science and Medicine*, 58: 2171–9.
Gilleard, C. and Higgs, P. (2000) *Cultures of Ageing*. Harlow: Pearson Education.
Gilleard, C., Higgs, P., Hyde, M., Wiggins, R. and Blane, D. (2005) 'Class, cohort, and consumption: the British experience of the third age', *Journal of Gerontology*, 60B(6): S305–10.
Laslett, P. (1989) *A Fresh Map of Life: The Emergence of the Third Age*. London: Weidenfeld and Nicholson.
Rowe, J. and Kahn, R. (1998) *Successful Aging*. New York: Dell.

I. C.

The social organization of death and dying

Over the past century, there have been considerable changes in the ways that western societies have approached the subject of death and dying. These changes in the social meanings attached to death and dying have been shaped by a range of social processes, the outcomes of which has seen death become much less of a shared community experience and more one of personal and private grief (an outcome termed by sociologists as the 'privatization' of death). The social processes identified as contributing to this shift are outlined below:

- A decline in public exposure to death and dying;
- A decline in the culture of public mourning;
- The medicalization of death and dying;
- Achieving a 'good death'.

A DECLINE IN PUBLIC EXPOSURE TO DEATH AND DYING

What is known as the 'epidemiological transition' marks the historical shift from infectious epidemics being the primary cause of mortality within a population, to degenerative diseases such as cancers and heart disease becoming the primary cause. Death (during early childhood) from cholera, smallpox, diphtheria, tuberculosis, and many other infectious conditions was a characteristic of all industrial societies up until the development of public health interventions. These developments in sanitation, the provision of clean water supplies, and the building of less overcrowded housing occurred in the UK after the middle of the nineteenth century. These interventions together with a general rise in the standard of living led to dramatic increases in life expectancy for all (see **The life course**). As a consequence of this 'epidemiological transition', death now occurs primarily at the end (not the beginning) of life.

A DECLINE IN THE CULTURE OF PUBLIC MOURNING

This process in part also reflects a decline in the *sacred* in relation to the experience of death within modern secular societies. Death has gradually come to be perceived as separated from life with a commensurate shift in the corporeal (body) boundaries (both symbolic and actual) between the dead and the living. The majority of people now no longer see death as the gateway to a higher spiritual existence, but purely as the ending of biological life. This process has had important social consequences because of the limited opportunities for, and possible unacceptability of (within a fast-paced consumerist society), taking time off from normal roles and responsibilities in order to grieve for the death of friends and loved ones.

These social and cultural changes have all contributed in their own way to modern anxieties associated with a denial of death (Giddens, 1990).

THE MEDICALIZATION OF DEATH AND DYING

Following Illich's (1976) **medicalization** of life thesis which asserts that more and more aspects of daily life have been brought into the biomedical sphere of influence, there is an argument that modern hospitals reflect the institutional expression of a modern desire to 'contain' sickness and death and remove it from the public gaze. From this perspective the function of hospitals is to manage the 'technical aspects' of symptom control for those who are dying. The following two quotations illustrate this perspective:

> Never before have people died as noiselessly and hygienically as today. . . and never in social conditions so much fostering solitude. (Elias, 1985: 85)

> The medicalisation of society has brought the epoch of natural death to an end. . . the doctor, rather than the patient, struggles with death. (Illich, 1976: 210)

It is argued, that the logic of **The biomedical model of health** generates the illusion that death can somehow be controlled, since disease causes death and in theory all diseases can be conquered. However, because dying is regarded as an aspect of illness, then the 'sick role' may be seen to apply to such patients. As a result, the dying patient may be stigmatized in that they become perceived as being 'bad' patients because they are non-responsive to medical intervention. This process may manifest itself in avoidance of, and withdrawal from that patient by health professionals. Glaser and Strauss (1968) argued that the institutional setting of the hospital served to reduce the emotion, uncertainty and social tensions surrounding death and dying. This was achieved through the establishment of a regular and routine pattern of death for large numbers of patients. These professional norms and practices gave shape to an 'institutionalized dying process' which was constructed in order to avoid social disruption. The term 'dying' was used as a predictive term in clinical practice, allowing all those involved in the care of the dying patient to determine what to do, and what to feel, next.

ACHIEVING A 'GOOD DEATH'

Glaser and Strauss's social research was concerned with the ways in which the 'social order' of the hospital was managed to cope with the 'disruptive threat' to staff represented by caring for terminally ill patients. They posed the following moral question:

> Is it really proper, some people have asked, to deny a dying person the opportunity to make his peace, with his conscience and with his god, to settle his affairs and provide for the future of his family, and control his style of dying, much as he controlled his style of living? (Glaser and Strauss, 1965: 6)

Glaser and Strauss's study was one of the first to critically draw attention to the fact that the need to always think in terms of clinical intervention and treatment had too often blinded the medical profession to attending to the needs of the dying patient. Since then, a critical understanding of medicine's role deploying constructs such as 'over-treatment' and 'heroic medicine' has gradually emerged. This more critical understanding has led onto the development of such ideas as the notion of the 'Good Death'. Kellehear's (1990) work has been particularly influential in setting out an ideal-type of the 'good death' to be drawn upon by health professionals to support their practice, and against which descriptions of the actual dying experience of an individual can be set. The five features of the good death identified by Kellehear are:

1 Awareness of dying: A personal and social process of greater openness about the prognosis of an illness where it is known that there is a high probability of death.
2 Personal preparations and social adjustments, or what he termed the settling of 'emotional accounts'.
3 Public preparations: sorting out wills, putting practical affairs in order.
4 The relinquishing, where appropriate, of formal work roles. Too often it is automatically assumed that dying individuals are beyond the age of retirement, which would not be the case in relation to AIDS and forms of cancer.
5 A good death involves formal and informal farewells.

Professional attitudes towards dying have changed considerably over the past 20 years, influenced not only by the work of people like Kellehear, but also by a progressive shift in public consciousness and the influence of the 'hospice movement' in establishing guidelines for the organization of the care for terminally ill patients within hospitals. There is now a greater emphasis placed on the emotional and psychological dimensions of the experience of dying in medical practice; this has become known as the 'palliative care' approach (Buckman, 1993).

REFERENCES AND FURTHER READING

Buckman, R. (1993) 'Communication in palliative care: a practical guide', in D. Doyle et al. (eds), *The Oxford Textbook of Palliative Medicine*. Oxford: OMP.
Clarke, D. (ed.) (1993) *The Sociology of Death*. Oxford: Blackwell.
Elias, N. (1985) *The Loneliness of the Dying*. Oxford: Blackwell.
Giddens, A. (1990) *The Consequences of Modernity*. Cambridge: Polity Press.
Glaser, B. and Strauss, A. (1965) *Awareness of Dying*. Chicago: Aldine.
Glaser, B. and Strauss, A. (1968) *Time for Dying*. Chicago: University of Chicago Press.
Illich, I. (1976) *Limits to Medicine*. Harmondsworth: Pelican.
Kellehear, A. (1990) *Dying of Cancer: The Final Year of Life*. London: Harwood Academic Publisher.

I. C.

the social organization of death and dying

Part 3
Health Protection

Social inequalities in health

Health inequalities are an enduring and notable feature of modern global society. The chances and opportunities to lead a healthy, active and rewarding life free of illness and pain are not evenly distributed across and between societies. To take the example of social class difference in health outcomes, within the United Kingdom, a male from the lowest socio-economic group can on average expect to live 7.2 years less than a man from the highest social-economic group. The difference for women is slightly less at 5 years. Sometimes the difference can be much more marked. In the United Kingdom one of the lowest life expectancies can be found in the deprived Calton area of Glasgow where average male life expectancy there is 54 years. This low number of years compares poorly with the average male life expectancy of 80 in the more affluent nearby Lenzie area of Glasgow, and the 62-year average male life expectancy in India (WHO, 2008).

In just about all causes of morbidity and early mortality a clear class gradient exists; those at the lower end of society exhibit higher levels of ill health and premature death than those at the higher end of society. These distinct social patterns exist demonstrating that experiencing good or bad health does not necessarily relate to lifestyle choices or engaging in risk behaviours, such as smoking, drinking and eating fatty foods. It is rather where one is located by gender, ethnicity and social class, and in which country one lives that exert the greatest influences on one's health. This perspective is very much in line with the **social model of health** that stresses that health is much more than understanding the normal or abnormal functioning of biological systems. Over the years, numerous reports and evidence have explored and confirmed how gender, ethnicity and class influence morbidity, mortality and self-perceived health. Reports such as *The Black Report* and *The Acheson Inquiry* and more recently the World Health Organization's (CSDH 2008) *Closing the Gap in a Generation* all share similar conclusions: that health inequalities are a very real and demonstrable feature of health in society, and that the reason for them continuing to exist are social and not individual in origin.

These social causes of health inequalities are evident in the vast amount of research in this area. It is the effects of income inequality, the

social inequalities in health

61

distribution of resources and political power, living in a fragmented and divided society, racism and the performance of gender that we should explore in order to understand why such inequalities exist. Often these processes are subtle and complex in how they operate and exert an influence on people's health. Taking class and health inequalities as an example once more, it is not just having a lack of nutritious food or living in sub-standard accommodation that negatively conditions health. Important as these considerations are, subtle and, perhaps, less obvious issues are also at play. The psycho-social strain, the chronic emotional stress, for example, of being alienated from other people and not being able to exert control in the workplace and other spheres of life can have just as damaging effects. Trying to cope with these strains can also explain why people from lower social economic groups tend to have higher levels of smoking and alcohol use. As Bartley (2003: 20) points out, such behaviours should be perceived as being a response to 'dull the experiences of uncertainty and isolation'.

The experience of direct and indirect racism is an important reason to explain why people from ethnic minority groups report worse health than white majority groups in the UK. For many people from ethnic minority groups, racism in its many forms can be a common and daily experience. Racism can, for example, be experienced on a structural level, with people from ethnic minority groups being more likely to be found in low-income employment leading to the risk of poverty and the attendant poor health that it creates. Or racism can be experienced as daily intimidation and name calling, leading to a rise in chronic stress levels and the damaging implications that entail for psycho-social health. Even though class, gender and ethnicity are the main axis of health inequality, care should be taken not to regard each inequality as belonging to a separate domain. Often the various inequalities intersect and influence each other creating further levels and forms of health disadvantage. So, for example, working-class people from ethnic minority groups are more likely to experience worse health than their middle-class peers from the same ethnic group, while women from ethnic groups are more likely to report having worse health than men from ethnic groups.

Health inequalities also raise challenging moral and ethical questions. Essentially, health inequalities emerge out of social, economic and cultural processes. As such, there is nothing inevitable or 'natural' about their occurrence, and since they are social in origin, it should be within the power of society to establish health *equality*. The health inequalities research importantly reveals significant numbers of people whether on a global basis or in a distinct nation-state, whose lives and overall well-being are not (and sometimes this is a considerable difference) as long or as fulfilling as others. A common theme in all international human rights charters and most national human rights legislation is that people are entitled to and should expect to lead a healthy life that is free of physical and emotional suffering. Two consequences follow from these statements.

First, and on a philosophical level, is it morally justifiable that people should have their lives negatively affected by poor health because of circumstances beyond their control? Second, if we do accept a moral duty to tackle health inequalities, what should governments, who are charged with ensuring the human rights of their citizens, do to reduce or even eradicate health inequalities?

Possible answers to these questions raise profound issues about contemporary societies that go beyond just focusing on health. Inequality is a general and distinctive feature of western society and is reproduced by the various economic, social and cultural structures of those societies. Other examples of inequality are evident in education, housing, income and political power, for example. Tackling health inequalities may therefore require addressing fundamentals of western capitalist societies. Even 'modest' reforms raise difficult political and economic challenges. Mitchell et al. (2000) claim that 11,509 lives could be saved in the United Kingdom if wealth inequalities were reduced to their 1983 levels, there was an end to child poverty and the creation of full employment. Achieving such aims would have all manner of implications for taxation and social policy, possibly requiring a substantial redistribution of wealth, a policy that might not be accepted by powerful interest groups who wish to maintain the status quo as it benefits their social position. Then again, a possible counterargument could claim that by improving the overall health of a population, a net gain in wealth for the economy as a whole can be realized, as a healthy workforce is more productive than an unhealthy workforce and therefore good for the economy. Such an ambition partly animated the founding of the British welfare state at the end of the Second World War, which sought to bring about both a fairer and more equal society

social inequalities in health

REFERENCES AND FURTHER READING

Bartley, M. (2003)*Health Inequality: An Introduction to Theories, Concepts and Methods.* Bristol: The Polity Press.
CSDH (World Health Organization) (2008) *Closing the Gap in a Generation: health equity through action on the social determinants of health. Final Report of the Commission on Social Determinants of Health.* Geneva: World Health Organization.

Mitchell, R., Shaw, M. and Dorling, D. (2000) *Inequalities in Life and Death: What if Britain Were More Equal?* Bristol: The Polity Press.

WHO (World Health Organization) (2008) *Key Concepts*. Available at: http://www.who.int/social_determinants/thecommission/finalreport/key_concepts/en/ (Accessed September 2009).

C. Y.

Social capital

Fine (2001) makes the accurate observation that 'social capital', next to globalization, is one of the most commonly cited, debated and researched concepts in the social sciences. As a concept, social capital has recently enjoyed an almost meteoric rise from an obscure article by Robert Putnam, a leading developer of and author on social capital theory, to being an important element in governmental and departmental policy. Most significantly, the World Bank has adopted the promotion of social capital in many of its social improvement schemes and policies as a mechanism to increase the well-being of people in low-income communities and nations.

Part of the appeal of social capital is that it is a reasonably straightforward concept at root, and, in many ways, speaks to already existing social science notions of community, mutual aid and the benefits of collaborative working with other people. Put very simply, social capital means that if people co-operate and engage in helpful reciprocal relationships in which they feel some form of emotional attachment (particularly trust and respect) then all manner of good outcomes for individuals, communities and societies will follow. Advocates of social capital have claimed that where high levels of social capital exist, then there are improvements in education, the economy, in lowering crime rates and, of course, in improving health. The conceptual origins of social capital are sketched out below, followed by more detail on the concept, before concluding with a brief summary of criticisms of the concept that have been made.

The concept of social capital is most commonly associated with Robert Putnam (2000) and his monograph *Bowling Alone*. His central claim is that American society is worse off now than it was back in the 1950s and 1960s because of a decline in social capital. He points to how American social life in that period was characterized by high membership of clubs, societies and other forms of civic engagement, such as the bowling leagues, emblematic in his work for the decline of social capital. Americans in the 1950s were much more motivated to associate and engage with others as opposed to leading the individualized existence that people experience today. The central image Putnam deploys in the book is of ten-pin bowling. Even though many, if not more, Americans go bowling today, it is as an individual (hence bowling alone) and not as a member of a league as was the case in the 1950s. Without participating in a league, Putnam argues, the crucial relationships with other people, and all the individual and communal benefits that these may bring, are absent. Putnam blames television as being the main culprit responsible for corroding ties between people, leading to a more individualized society.

As suggested above, social capital shares common ground with existing traditions in the social sciences. Even though Putnam is widely associated with introducing the concept of social capital, other theorists and social scientists have included the basic tenets of social capital in their work, though not always using the term social capital (Farr, 2004). In classical sociology, the notion of people working and co-operating together for their mutual advancement is found in the philosophical writings of Marx. Durkheim also visits this idea in his meditations on social solidarity and the requirement for people to engage with each other in order for a society to function effectively. More recently, the influential French sociology Pierre Bordieu used the term 'social capital' to analyze the connections among the business elites, and how, alongside other forms of capital, that assisted in the reproduction of social distinctions and hierarchies.

Social capital is not a unitary phenomenon. Rather, it is manifest in different forms in relation to the types of people and social groups who are co-operating. *Bonding* capital refers to groups of people who all share certain common characteristics. These groups can be exclusive and unwilling to admit members who do not share the traits of that particular group. *Bridging* capital, on the other hand, refers to a more inclusive form of social capital, where people from a diversity of backgrounds join together to participate in mutually beneficial networks. The relationships between those involved in bridging capital tend to be less strong than those found in bonding capital. It is bridging social capital this is reckoned to be the

social capital

most effective in producing the positive outcomes that social capital can apparently bring. Putnam (2000: 19) pithily summarizes the differences between the two as, 'bonding social capital constitutes a kind of sociological glue, whereas bridging social capital provides a sociological WD40'. Ultimately, however, both have to operate in parallel: bonding capital bringing groups of people together in a locality or community, with bridging capital bringing those groups together on a regional or national basis. There are, therefore, vertical and horizontal aspects to social capital.

The small US town of Roseto in the state of Pennsylvania is often advanced as an example of how social capital can be beneficial for health. In many respects it is not dissimilar to many other small towns in America, save for two interesting aspects. First, it has had for much of its history much better health, especially in relation to heart disease, than neighbouring towns of broadly similar population size and low income. Second, Roseto has received the attentions of a variety of medical and sociological researchers over time attempting to establish why that health advantage existed. The main reason that was established by the researchers for the town's good health lay with the tight-knit nature of the Italian-American community. As a community, they maintained the culture of strong civic engagement inherited from the region of Italy from where most of the original migrants had left for America. All three generations would eat together, if not with neighbours, at mealtimes, while membership of civic, secular and religious societies was common, as were town-wide fetes and galas. Additionally, and importantly, there was very little emphasis on displays of wealth or of being more successful than one's fellow Rosetans. Being part of the community was more important than any sense of individuality. Crucially, throughout the 1980s onwards, the community became increasingly culturally American, losing sight of their more communal Italian roots and becoming more individualized in their personal and public lives. This decline in civic engagement saw Roseto's health advantage considerably lessen. This reduction in good health occurred in spite of the town's inhabitants becoming wealthier. (Wolf and Bruhn, 1993)

It is the support that social capital can offer that appears to be the reason why a relationship between high social capital and good health exists (see **Social inequalities in health**). That support can either be instrumental or affective. Instrumental support is the providing of information, checking up on older or vulnerable individuals in the community, or perhaps just hurrying someone along to the doctor if they are looking unwell. Affective support relates to emotions and helping people through bad or stressful times in their lives. Evidence exists that strongly indicates a link between on-going chronic stress and poor mental and physical health. Support can therefore act as buffer against the worst effects of stressful events, thereby reducing any potential negative health effects.

As with any concept, social capital has attracted criticism. Portes (1998) and Fine (2001) have criticized social capital for being far too loose and diverse a concept. As a consequence of this lack of precision, just about anything can be termed 'social capital', if it appears to bring people together. Navarro (2004) has noted that social capital may be good for the health of some people but their social capital and well-being are built on the exploitation of others. Muntaner et al. (2002) have upbraided social capital theory in two ways. First, it can be used to blame communities where high levels of poor health exist for having low levels of social capital, which takes attention away from inadequate social policy in providing appropriate housing, suitable health care and high standards of education. Second, working-class examples of social capital networks, such as trade unions, are often absent in measures of social capital as sociologists tend to prefer middle-class examples of social capital networks.

Social capital has established itself as one of the most pre-eminent concepts in health and social policy. Its appeal to community and bringing people together are two of its main aspects. The application and influence of social capital will no doubt be noted for some time to come. In terms of Health Studies, it is an important concept to explore and understand both in terms of what its supporters and critics have to say.

REFERENCES AND FURTHER READING

Farr, J. (2004) 'Social capital: an intellectual history', *Political Theory*, 31(1): 6–33.

Fine, B. (2001) *Social Capital Theory Versus Social Theory: Political Economy And Social Science at the Turn of the Millennium*. London: Routledge.

Halpern, D. (2005) *Social Capital*. Cambridge: Polity.

Muntaner, C., Lynch, J. W., Hillemeier, M., Lee, J. H., David, R., Benach, J. and Borrell, C. (2002) 'Economic inequality, working-class power, social capital and cause-specific mortality on wealthy countries', *International Journal of Health Services*, 32(4): 629–56.

National Statistics (2006) *Focus on Health*. Hampshire: Palgrave Macmillan.

Navarro, V. (2004) 'Commentary: Is capital the solution or the problem?' *International Journal of Epidemiology*, 33(4): 672–4.

Portes, A. (1998) 'Social capital: its origins and applications in modern sociology', *Annual Review of Sociology*, 24: 1–24.

Putnam, R. D. (2000) *Bowling Alone: The Collapse and Revival of Social Capital in Contemporary Society*. New York: Simon & Schuster.

Wolf, S. and Bruhn, S. G. (1993) *The Power of Clan: The Influence of Human Relationships on Heart Disease*. Brunswick: Transaction.

C. Y.

social capital

Risk society

The late-modern societies that we live within now possess the technological and material resources to potentially identify and manage many forms of 'risk' (to health, to profit, to the environment) that hitherto had been beyond any form of control. This new 'risk culture' (Beck, 1992) has resulted in a much greater awareness of the extent of 'risk' within society. This 'reflexive modernism' reflects the shift from ignorance or private fears about the unknown to a widespread knowledge about the world we have created. Within the 'risk society', knowledge of risks has 'become the motor of the self-politicisation of modernity' (Beck, 1992: 181). However, 'risk awareness' has consequences for both society and for individuals, for even though risk has always been a feature of human life and society, in late-modern society the perception of risk has increasingly become disproportionate to the 'actual' consequences of risk. Despite huge advances in the understanding of disease risks, the media over the past decade or so have regularly reported health scare stories concerning 'Mad Cow' disease, MMR vaccinations, and the risks posed by bird and swine flu, to name but a few.

Sociologists Beck (1992) and Giddens (1999) have argued that we now live in a 'risk society', a society where much societal and individual attention is focused on avoiding and managing risk. The risks that cause concern are also of a different form than in previous epochs. While pre-modern societies faced risks that were external (famines, floods and droughts, for example), late-modern societies have to tackle manufactured risks, potential problems that have been created by our own technologies and industries. Current concerns with the environment are an example of this trend where human industrialization has led to a vast array of potential problems for the planet and for human society.

Crucial to understanding risk within contemporary society is that 'risk' is not simply people acting rationally (or not), according to well-informed expert opinion and advice. It is, rather, how people and society are changed by the prominence of risk in so many aspects of everyday life. After all, not all risks are actually 'real', and sometimes the avoidance of what is deemed to be a risk leads to a worse outcome than what would have occurred had the risk not been defined as such in the first place. To explore these issues further, a brief summary of how 'risk society' has emerged and how it has changed both people and society is undertaken next.

It was scarcity of the basics of life, natural disaster and a fear of God's wrath that figured largely in the minds of people in feudal and pre-modern times. A secure material basis that could provide all the basics (and some of the luxuries) of life was not possible then. Existence was very much hand-to-mouth and highly precarious for most of the population. A summer drought or a bad harvest could mean starvation and possibly death. Life was therefore to be lived in the present with little thought to what could lie ahead. The world at this time was also informed and understood in religious terms. Every aspect of life inescapably carried some form of religious element. Plough Monday, the first day back at work after the Christmas holidays involved the local priest blessing farmyard tools, for example, before work could begin. This all-encompassing religious worldview also gave rise to the fear that the Apocalypse was imminent and that eternal damnation was not that far away. In these pre-modern times risk was beyond human control, up to the whims of nature and to God's will.

This situation is in very much marked contrast with modern societies. From the Enlightenment in the mid-eighteenth century onwards, humanity has sought to be in charge of its own destiny. Rational objective science has provided people with a different understanding of both nature and of the supernatural. Humans can now, in certain, but not all, societies possess the means to overcome the problems and risks posed by scarce material resources. Food, warmth and shelter are obtainable for the majority in a population. For those who do not possess such resources, it is not because they are intrinsically scarce. There are, for example, surplus houses but yet homelessness exists. Any scarcity is due to social norms and practices and not because there is an insufficient supply of a needed resource. Droughts and bad harvests are therefore not the risk they once were, though such external risks do pose issues for certain populations in low-income countries. With scarcity no longer an issue, the living for today mentality of pre-modern times has been replaced by a modern mindset that can think and plan ahead. Human activity is now directed to the future and how we can best realize our well-being. Identifying, managing and avoiding risk becomes part of that perspective. These historical developments would suggest that a safe risk-free world should have been created, yet the technological advances that were made created new forms of risk that were quite inconceivable to previous generations.

It is how risk changes and alters the perceptions and actions of individuals and societies that is of interest for Health Studies. So if religion informed the daily experiences of people in pre-modern times then the anticipation

risk society

of risk may inform the daily experiences of people in late-modernity. Everyday activity is infused with notions of risk. For example, take sitting down at a desk in order to work using a computer. Such a simple activity is now potentially exposed to all manner of risks, such as repetitive strain injury or pulled back muscles and a variety of health risks, for instance. These risks are now subject to intervention on a structural societal level in the form of health and safety legislation, but also on an individual level. The office worker has now to ensure that they are sitting correctly and have arranged their desk in a manner that will reduce the risk of anything bad happening to them. There is also a moral dimension to risk implied in this example. The 'good' citizen in late-modernity is one who is risk-aware and who does their uppermost to avoid risk. These good works of risk avoidance are evident in eating low-fat foods or taking exercise, for example.

Risk society puts experts in a paradoxical position. On one hand, the sheer complexity of modern life almost requires people to turn to experts for information and guidance, and as new risks are identified, new information is therefore needed. Experts are not accorded the same deference as they were formerly, however. People may judge expert advice in the context of other social actors who are also providing information on the risk, or may just decide for themselves. The MMR (Measles, Mumps and Rubella) vaccination controversy in the United Kingdom provides an example of this trend. What Hobson-West (2007) noted was that parents did not always accept – if not reject outright – dominant expert discourses of vaccination. They tended to reject the advice of official bodies that stressed immunization had to be thought of in terms of being society-wide to have any effect, to achieve what epidemiologists refer to as herd immunity where between 85 to 90 per cent of a population are immunized. The parents in this case opted for individual solutions, assessing the risks for their own children as opposed to taking account of the wider implications. The main consequence was that by lowering the overall number of immunized children, the risk of an individual child contracting measles, mumps or rubella could actually increase.

Over-emphasizing risk is the final aspect of risk society to be considered here. The increased emphasis on risks leads to the identification of more and more causes of risk. This activity can cause something that was formerly considered benign now to be a source of risk and therefore the object of risk management and avoidance. As a consequence, perceptions of risk can be highly selective or partial, leading to panics and health scares. Christakis (2008) comments that the perceived risk of health problems as a consequence of food allergies, in particular, peanut allergies, is disproportionate to the numbers of people who actually suffer an adverse reaction. He notes that of 3.3 million Americans, only 150 adults and children die each year from *all* food allergies combined. This figure should be compared against the 10,000 children admitted to hospitals from brain injuries sustained from sports injuries, yet it is the humble peanut that is seen as a major threat to health rather than the sports field. The over-reaction to the risks of peanut allergy has seen parents making their children's lives a 'peanut-free zone'. Once again, this can actually have the opposite effect to the one intended with children more, rather than less, likely to develop a food allergy.

REFERENCES AND FURTHER READING

Beck, U. (1992) *Risk Society: Towards a New Modernity*. London: Sage.
Christakis, N. A. (2008) 'This allergies hysteria is just nuts', *BMJ*, 337: a2880.
Giddens, A. (1999) *Runaway World: How Globalization is Reshaping Our Lives*. London: Profile.
Hobson-West, P. (2007) 'Trusting blindly can be the biggest risk of all: organised resistance to childhood vaccination in the UK', *Sociology of Health and Illness*, 29(3):

C. Y.

Public health

Achieving good health in a population is often said to, 'rest largely on shaping the distribution of risk in a population (see **Risk society**) so that fewer people are exposed to risky situations' (Berkman and Melchoir, 2006: 55). Effective interventions to reduce risk at a population level can only ever be coordinated and delivered by government (or more properly, 'the State') as only it has the resources and (political) responsibility to limit the 'excesses' (or 'externalities' as they are sometime termed) of the market economy that give rise (both directly and indirectly) to so many of these health risks. However, public health and preventative health policies, which can be defined as action taken at a societal level in order to protect and promote the health of the whole population, have traditionally constituted only a marginal place in the activity and funding of health care systems, including the NHS. The influence of the biomedical causality model of ill health has been a major contributory factor in the failure to adequately address the social and environmental factors which shape ill health at a population level. The average proportion of spending on public health is just 2.9 per cent of total health care budgets in developed (OECD) countries (OECD, 2005).

The first initiatives to achieve better levels of health for the population that established the basis of state intervention in Britain were the Public Health Acts of the mid-nineteenth century. This legislation was primarily concerned with improving sanitation and housing in the newly industrialized towns and cities where infectious disease epidemics were common and a direct consequence of the lack of clean water supplies, overcrowding and poverty, and resulted in unprecedented levels of mortality, particularly among the very young. The 1848 Public Health Act created a national Board of Health, and gave towns the right to appoint a Medical Officer of Health, while the 1875 Act enforced laws about slum clearance, provision of sewers and clean water, and the removal of nuisances. The benefits of these measures soon became clear to all, as rates of infectious disease began to drop significantly, so that, by the late nineteenth century, towns and city corporations (incipient local authorities) were competing with one another to provide the best level of public health for their citizens (and this was at a time well before germ theory had established that micro-organisms were the cause of most infectious diseases). As an illustration of this point, death rates (mortality) from respiratory tuberculosis (TB) fell from 4,000 deaths per million of the population in 1838 down to 500 per million by the 1930s.

McKeown (1979) in his classic work on the origins of public health, identified the major factors in the decline in mortality from infectious diseases as being these general improvements in nutrition and sanitation that occurred from the mid-nineteenth century onwards. These measures improved individual resistance to, and reduced the spread of, infectious diseases. Although medical science had the capability by the end of that century to identify the causative agent, effective treatments were not available until the mid-twentieth century. Hence, by the time that immunization and vaccination programmes had been developed for many of these infectious diseases, their impact on reducing mortality was limited, given the enormous improvement in the general standard of living that had occurred. Yet these first large-scale infrastructural improvements to reduce the threat to the health of the population as a whole were not built upon, and public health initiatives after the 1880s came to be focused at the level of the individual citizen with the development of immunization programmes as well as a particular obsession with personal hygiene. The rise of hospital-based therapeutic medicine in the early twentieth century tended to weaken the role of local public health departments, and this situation did not change with the inception of the National Health Service in 1946 after the Second World War.

It was not until over a century after the first Public Health Acts that there was to be a return to focusing on environmental change (in addition to personal prevention measures) as central to any public health strategy. What came to be called the 'New Public Health' (NPH) Movement emerged in the 1970s as a response to the apparent failures of the biomedical therapeutic approach to effectively improve the health of the population as a whole. This approach embraced the broad vision of the mid-nineteenth-century legislation that had recognized that population health risks lay in environmental and social structural factors beyond the control of individuals themselves. The NPH movement gradually became established across North America and Western Europe and has been influential in shaping the World Health Organization's *Global Health Strategy* (WHO, 1981) and the European regional strategy (WHO, 1985). Nevertheless, while at the level of supra-national health organizations, these ideas concerning the object of public health gained credence, particularly in relation to interventions in the developing world, at the levels of national government (and particularly within the UK reflecting the general underfunding of health care at that time), there was little enthusiasm for direct legislative interventions to curb the new environmental threats to health.

One of the most eminent and influential critics of this individualized approach to public health was the epidemiologist Geoffrey Rose (1992), who described this clinically-oriented approach as a 'high-risk strategy' to prevention. Rose drew on the understanding that there exists a social distribution of exposure to causative risk factors to develop an argument for assessing and tackling what were seen to be primarily individual behavioural determinants of the health at the societal level. His work demonstrated that rather than identifying those individuals who are living with a particular disease (with an associated causative health risk exposure) as being somehow in a different category than the rest of the 'normal' population (in line with the biomedical model), we should see them as just one end of a population continuum. One of the examples Rose cites to demonstrate this point is the phenomenon of high blood pressure (hypertension).

People with hypertension are not a distinct group separate from a normal distribution of blood pressure in society, they do not have a specific defect not present in the bulk of a population, but actually come within the range of variability described by a bell curve of a normal statistical distribution. After examining the distribution of risk factors for hypertension in a number of different countries at various levels of economic development, Rose concluded that the proportion of people at high risk in any population is simply a function of the *average* blood pressure, cholesterol levels, etc., in that particular society. These conclusions concerning the social distribution and determinants of disease cut across the notion of disease as an 'autonomous individual affliction'. His alternative 'population strategy' sought to shift the population distribution of a risk factor as a more effective strategy to reduce the burden of disease in a society than targeting people at high risk. It emphasizes that modern diseases and the exposure to the range of causative risk factors are a product of the norms of any particular society.

However, Rose's approach, which essentially advocated changes in the physical and social structure in order to reduce the population disease burden, has never been adopted by any government. Public health strategies within the UK continue to be largely dominated by strategies designed to promote individual disease risk factor modification (see **Health promotion**).

REFERENCES AND FURTHER READING

Berkman, L. and Melchoir, M. (2006) 'The shape of things to come: how social policy impacts social integration and family structure to produce population health', in J. Siegrist and M. Marmot (eds), *Social Inequalities in Health: New Evidence and Policy Implications*. Oxford: Oxford University Press, pp 55–72.

Lomas, J. (1998) 'Social capital and health: Implications for public health and epidemiology', *Social Science and Medicine*, 47(9): 1181–8.

McKeown, T. (1979) *The Role of Medicine – Dream, Mirage or Nemesis* – Part 1, Oxford: Basil Blackwell.

OECD (2005) *Health at a Glance: OECD Indicators 2005*. Paris: OECD.

Rose, G. (1992) *The Strategy of Preventive Medicine*. Oxford: Oxford University Press.

WHO (World Health Organization) (1981) *Global Health Strategy for All by the Year 2000*. Geneva: WHO.

WHO (World Health Organization) (1985) *Targets for Health for All*. Copenhagen: Regional Office for Europe.

I. C.

Health promotion

Health promotion is concerned with providing people with the techniques, support networks and information in order to enable them to make positive changes to their health. As a health strategy it is essentially predicated on the assumptions of Humanistic philosophy (influenced in particular by Maslow's hierarchy of needs approach, as well as Carl Rogers' notion of the development of a self-concept). This is a philosophy which argues that, given the correct social environment, social networks, and the requisite knowledge, individuals possess both the capacity and the human right to facilitate better health for themselves.

The need for substantial changes in population health is necessary due to the existence and persistence of health inequalities both on a national or global scale. As Jong-wook, Director-General of the World Health Organization (2003: 2083) has commented, 'Inequalities scar the world's health landscape.' Far too many people have their lives shortened or their well-being compromised by unnecessary poor health. There is nothing "natural" or unavoidable about such inequalities existing, they result from social, historical and cultural conditions (see **Social inequalities in health**). Health promotion is frequently presented as a strategy that could help to reverse unequal health outcomes. This entry on health promotion therefore outlines the main ideas behind health promotion in addition to identifying some formidable challenges that health promotion encounters.

The strategy of health promotion shares many of the tenets of the social model of health (see **The social model of health**), in recognizing the multidimensional nature of health for a given population. This commitment to a rounded and holistic conception of health is evident in the Ottawa Charter (WHO, 1986), a key health promotion document that has influenced policy on a global and national level. The central approaches the charter envisages for realizing the aims of health promotion are as follows (WHO, 1986: 2–3):

- That all policy, and not just specific health policies, should take issues of health into account and be focused on promoting good health.
- To build supportive and cohesive networks between and with communities as good health emerges out of such relationships.

- To allow communities to have a greater say and greater control in what affects them.
- To support the development of personal life skills in order to enhance an individual's capacity to make decisions that are good for their health.
- To move the emphasis of health services away from treating the ill and the sick to creating and maintaining a healthy society.
- To create an equal society that allows everyone to realize their potential and in doing so become healthier.

The Ottawa Charter also outlines three concepts by which effective health promotion should work. The first is *advocacy*, which requires health promotion to push and highlight the need for health in all areas of life. The next is *enablement*, which calls for the creation of the circumstances for all people (regardless of class, gender or ethnicity) to have as much control over their lives as possible. Finally, to *mediate* between various social groups in government, business and the wider community in order to coordinate policy, strategies and activities that lead to a healthier society.

In the UK, the focus of health promotion has changed considerably over time. The earlier examples of health promotion were orientated towards disease and infection prevention with individuals being very much the recipients of expert advice and government direction. Contemporary health promotion has shifted away from this 'top-down' approach and is now more likely to embrace 'bottom-up' approaches – though sometimes 'older' perspectives are still used in practice, particularly in medical settings. The emphasis is firmly on active partnership and involving people in decision-making and planning. This shift entails the health professional working in partnership as opposed to instructing the people with whom they are working. In parallel to this focus on participation is a move away from concentrating on individuals at risk from specific diseases to thinking in terms of the population as a whole. In fact, as is summarized in the entry on **global health**, perspectives on improving health are moving further towards thinking about the world's population as opposed to the population of a particular nation-state.

However, as with any other attempt to introduce behaviour change, health promotion faces some very distinct, if not formidable, challenges. Structural versus individual influences on health provide one distinct tension. Nevertheless, the strategy of health promotion has been criticized for offering an over-individualized approach to health, even though a rhetorical commitment to a social perspective of health may exist, too often health promotion campaigns have been primarily concerned to identify so-called 'problem' or 'at-risk' groups, such as adolescent drug-users, pregnant teenagers, smokers, the 'obese', and many more. Interventions are then directed at persuading these groups to change or control their behaviour or 'lifestyle' so as to reduce the damage they are perceived to be causing to their health through unprotected sex, smoking, unbalanced diet, etc. The underlying assumption is that it is individual volitional behaviour that constitutes the primary risk to health. Alternatively, raising substantial numbers of the population out of poverty would undoubtedly lead to substantial improvements to thousands of people's health, yet this would require a public commitment by government to a sizable financial investment and potentially contentious social policies such as wealth redistribution; so far this has not occurred.

What may appear to be a sensible and logical health message in the context of one person's life circumstances may not be feasible or achievable for others. The context of someone's life is shaped by the social structures of class, gender and ethnicity, as mentioned above. These structures affect people in obvious ways, for example, by limiting someone's ability to be able to purchase healthy food. They also influence people's lives in more subtle and possibly unexpected ways too. A useful example is provided by Graham's (1993) research on smoking among young lone-parent women. As a distinct social group they would be prime candidates for giving up smoking given their health needs and how little money with which they had to exist. This, however, was not the case. For the women, smoking was perceived as one of the few 'luxuries' and sources of solace in an otherwise frantic, demanding and complex life. Stopping smoking would have entailed abandoning one of the few pleasures they had in life.

Health promotion strategies seek to achieve better health for all. Whilst this is a potentially achievable and worthwhile aim, trying to realize this goal through individual behaviour-change alone without accompanying social structural change inevitably sets limits to the long-term impact of even well-resourced initiatives.

REFERENCES AND FURTHER READING

Graham, H. (1993) *When Life's a Drag: Women, Smoking and Disadvantage*. London: HMSO.

Jong-wook, L. (2003) 'Global improvement and WHO: shaping the future', *The Lancet*, 362(20/27): 2083–8.

WHO (World Health Organization) (1986) Ottawa Charter for Health Promotion. Available at: http://www.who.int/hpr/NPH/docs/ottawa_charter_hp.pdf.

C. Y./I. C.

Work and health

It has become a truism that modern societies are experiencing an 'epidemic' of work-related stress. Research to discover what the factors are that have precipitated this phenomenon are typically grounded in an epidemiological understanding of the causal relationship (using statistical measures of association between variables leading to particular patterns of health and disease outcome aggregated at a population level) that exists between work characteristics, psychological stress and ill health. This approach is reflected within the highly influential 'Demand-Control-Support' (DCS) model (Karasek and Theorell, 1990).

The DCS model proposes that job strain is likely to occur when a person faces the following: (a) *high job demands* in combination with (b) *low job control* and (c) *low social support* from colleagues and managers. The job control variable itself consists of two components: (i) 'decision authority', that is, being able to choose when and how tasks are completed, and (ii) skill discretion, defined as whether a job is boring or repetitive, and the extent to which skills can be used and developed.

The DCS job strain model seeks to provide quantitative data that can be correlated with indicators of psychological well-being and physical health. A key assumption of the model is that job stress variables are inherently pathogenic and that they can be separated from the personal attributes and characteristics of an individual worker. This model received considerable empirical support from the Whitehall II studies which examined the social inequalities that existed in mortality from coronary heart disease among different grades of UK civil servants (Marmot et al., 1991). The work of Bosma et al. (1997) which drew on the Whitehall II study data noted that lower control over choosing what to do at work, not having a say in planning, or not deciding work speed within working environment impacted negatively on health outcomes. Kivimaki et al. 's (2000) study of a large public organization in Finland experiencing a downsizing of the staff also examined the underlying mechanisms which produced a subsequent deterioration in the health of employees. The authors found that the increase in sickness absence was mediated not only by the heightened job insecurity but also by subsequent increase in job demands and a lowering of job control. While Cheng et al. (2000) in their study of the association between psychosocial work characteristics and health of 20,000 American nurses,

key concepts in
health studies

78

found that, '[T]he decline in health functioning associated with job strain were as large as those associated with smoking and sedentary lifestyles'.

A more critical understanding has argued that 'stress-related personal injury' is treated within the DCS model as an unmediated effect of objective work conditions. The underpinning assumption is that high job demands, low job control and low social support are inherently pathogenic in the same way that asbestos is carcinogenic. Social factors are treated as if they were objective pathogens that exercise their effect on the human organism regardless of the perceptions and beliefs of the worker. The variables assessed by the job strain model are primarily concerned with psychological stress, anxiety and depression embodied (or presenting themselves) as physical symptoms and therefore measurable as physiological changes. However, work stress experiences at work also crucially involve perception, cognition and reflection on the part of the individual; these psychosocial variables are not as straightforward to objectively measure. Therefore, the issue with an epidemiological understanding of work stress 'is not that the relationship between work characteristics and morbidity is spurious, but that it fails to grasp the role of consciousness in mediating that relationship' (Wainwright and Calnan, 2000: 231). By contrast, sociological and psychological approaches to examining the relationship between work stress experiences and health outcomes emphasize the ways in which social and cultural factors mediate hierarchical relationships in the workplace. The research focus is the factors which serve to enhance or diminish the resilience of the working population to demanding work characteristics.

One example of this sociological approach is Hochschild's (1983) classic study (*The Managed Heart*) of work-related stress amongst air stewardesses in the airline industry. The consciousness element that is missing from the DCS model is to some extent accounted for in Hochschild's study through the application of the concept of 'emotional labour' (or 'emotion management'). The study draws attention to the ways in which the emotions of air stewardesses are expropriated for profit, as their job requires that they produce a welcoming emotional environment for the airline's clientele. In doing so, they are required to draw upon both their physical and mental energies in addition to their deeper emotional core. For these air stewardesses, everyday social 'gestures of exchange' thus become commodified. Similar results have been found among other groups of workers required to provide this emotional element in their everyday work activities, such as nurses and other groups of care workers, and for all these groups the outcomes of emotional labour for personal health are quite considerable. Williams (1998: 754), commenting on Hochschild's study, observed that it was replete with references to the 'human costs' of emotional labour from 'burnout' to feeling 'phoney', from 'cynicism' to 'emotional deadness', 'guilt' to self 'blame'.

A strong correlation between the experience of work-related stress and poor health outcomes was highlighted within the Acheson Report (1998) commissioned by the New Labour government to examine social inequalities in health on coming into power more than a decade ago. The Department of Health's shift in an understanding of the importance of addressing work-related stress is set-out in the following excerpt taken from the current Public Health White Paper:

> [E]vidence has shown that poor working arrangements, such as lack of job control or discretion, consistently high work demands and low social support, can lead to musculoskeletal disorders, mental illness and sickness absence. The real task is to improve the quality of jobs by reducing monotony, increasing job control and applying HR practices and policies – organizations need to ensure that they adopt approaches that support the overall health and well-being of their employees. (DoH, 2004: 161)

REFERENCES AND FURTHER READING

Acheson Report (1998) *Independent Inquiry into Inequalities in Health.* London: The Stationery Office.

Bosma, H., Marmot, M., Hemingway, H., Nicholson, A., Brunner, E. and Stansfield, S. (1997) 'Low job control and the risk of coronary heart disease in Whitehall II (prospective cohort) study', *British Medical Journal*, 314: 558–65.

Cheng, Y., Kawachi, I., Coakley, E., Schwartz, J. and Colditz, G. (2000) 'Association between psychosocial work characteristics and health functioning in American women: prospective study', *British Medical Journal*, 320: 1432–6.

DoH (Department of Health) (2004) *Choosing Health: Making Healthy Choices Easier.* London: The Stationery Office.

Hochschild, A. (1983) *The Managed Heart: The Commercialisation of Human Feeling.* Berkeley, CA: University of California Press.

Karasek, R. and Theorell, T. (1990) *Healthy Work.* New York: Basic Books.

Kivimaki, M., Vahtera, J., Pentti, J. and Ferrie, J. (2000) 'Factors underlying the effect of organisational downsizing on health of employees: longitudinal cohort study', *British Medical Journal*, 320: 971–5.

Marmot, M., Smith, G., Stansfield, S. et al. (1991) 'Health inequalities among British civil servants – the Whitehall II study', *The Lancet*, 337: 1387–93.

Wainwright, D. and Calnan, M. (2000) 'Rethinking the work stress "epidemic"', *European Journal of Public Health*, 10: 231–4.

Williams, S. (1998) 'Modernity and the emotions: corporeal reflections on the (ir)rational', *Sociology*, 32(4): 747–69.

key concepts in
health studies

80

I. C.

Global health

Health, as so much of all aspects of twenty-first-century life, is inextricably bound up in global relationships. Global health therefore refers to perceiving health as the outcome of global processes, with solutions to improving the health of the global population as being the responsibility of an alliance of global organizations, national governments and non-governmental organizations.

The process of 'globalization' is an important feature of life in the twenty-first century, affecting and reordering many aspects of our personal lives and social interactions. In relation to economic, financial, cultural, and technological matters, as well as the mobility of its population, contemporary society is infused with relationships, symbols and products that lie beyond the immediacy of any specific nation-state. These outcomes of the process of globalization have led to a 'smaller' and, on many levels, more inter-dependent world. Decisions, events and developments in one country no longer only affect that locality but instead impinge upon, benefit and influence people in many different places and countries. Since so many other aspects of everyday life are now bound up to a greater and lesser extent with global impulses, it is appropriate too that health should be perceived similarly in global terms.

The concept of 'global health' therefore seeks to explore how health is increasingly conditioned and modulated by global processes and global relationships. A global health perspective conceives health as referring to the health of all the people on the planet. By adopting this perspective, which embraces the entire world, a radical break from the past was made when health initiatives were mainly focused on the health of people in one particular geographic region or specific population. It is also not just different groups of people around the world that global health brings under its auspices. The global approach to health, of bringing together different groups of people, is also apparent in other ways too. In terms of delivering global health, there is an acknowledgement of the roles and importance of different organizations and institutions. These varied organizations include national governments and non-governmental organizations (for example, Oxfam and the World Health Organization), influential private foundations (for example, the Soros Foundation) in addition to multinational corporations such as Microsoft. As well as bringing together a diversity of organizations, the study of global health also witnesses a bringing together of a diversity of academic disciplines. Insights from psychology, sociology, politics and social epidemiology are all mobilized to bring a fuller, richer and deeper understanding of the various dimensions of global health (Lee et al., 2002).

The WHO (2008) has identified the following challenges to health across the globe:

- One in five of the 58.8 million deaths that occurred in 2004 were children under the age of five. Malnutrition is one of the main reasons for those children dying.
- Lung cancer as a consequence of smoking is now the leading cause of cancer-related mortality for men.
- Ischemic heart disease and cardiovascular disease are the leading causes of death.
- HIV/AIDS is the main cause of death for 15–59-year-olds in the African region, accounting for 40 per cent of all female deaths.
- Depression and other instances of mental distress are among the leading causes of disability. Other causes of disability arise from vision and hearing impairments.
- Road traffic accidents are increasing globally due to increasing urbanization. Quite simply, more and more people are now living in built environments with greater proximity to cars, with all the advantages and disadvantages that entails.

However, these causes of death and disability are far from being equally distributed. A major task facing any global health strategy is to address the vast differences in health outcomes and life chances that exist both *between* and *in* countries. Life expectancy varies considerably around the world. For example, in high-income countries such as the UK, the USA and Japan, life expectancy is quite high at 79, 78 and 81, while in low-income countries life expectancy in Lesotho, Mozambique and Tanzania is 42, 50 and 50 respectively. Morbidity and mortality by specific disease vary quite markedly as well. The most notable example being that more people die of HIV/AIDS in Africa than of all causes in regions such as the high-income countries, the Americas and Western Pacific region (WHO, 2008). It is also important to note that health inequalities are also prevalent with*in* nation-states. The average life expectancy in the UK is 79; there are, however, sections of the British population that do not live that long. The variations are related to the social processes of class, ethnicity and gender (see **Social inequalities in health**).

What are the ways in which the process of globalization shapes health outcomes, and second, what global strategy could be enacted to bring about change? The SARS (Severe Acute Respiratory Syndrome) outbreak of 2003 that affected approximately 150 people worldwide provides a useful example of how health has become 'globalized' and how the very processes of globalization create new and complex health risks. The ease by which people can now travel conveniently and speedily around the world is one such key process of globalization. The means by which this ease of travel is made possible (cheap airfares, frequent flights, and a global network of air travel, for example) also provides the means by which disease can rapidly move from one country to the next. In this case, SARS, from its first identified outbreak in Hanoi, Vietnam, in February 2003, spread to Hong Kong, Thailand, Singapore and Canada in less than a month by 15 March 2003. The main reason for this rapid spread was people coming into contact with the syndrome in one country and then flying to another and transmitting it to other people on arrival. Basically, no ease of air travel, no rapid spread of SARS. This SARS example illustrates one mechanism by which globalization influences health. There are many other mechanisms that also exert an influence and are to do with the economic and trade relationships between high-income countries, such as the European nations and the USA, and low-income countries, especially in the Asian and African regions. These particular processes often function at the deeper structural levels in a society creating the conditions that either enable or inhibit the possibilities of good health. One useful example here is the activities of the World Trade Organization (WTO), the main forum for regulating world trade and again a key player in the various processes of globalization. As Ranson et al. (2002) argue, the WTO acts primarily to promote free trade between nation-states by reducing barriers to companies trading in other countries. In doing so, health may be adversely affected in a variety of ways. Local health regulatory regimes may have to be compromised to allow for free trade. By promoting free trade, other negative consequences could also follow. The actions of large multinational companies, for example, can depress workers' rights and earning potential, thus exacerbating income and social inequalities, an important cause of health inequalities (Wilkinson, 1996), and by making health care unaffordable for sections of the population.

The recent 2008 WHO publication, *Closing the Gap: Health Equity through Action on the Social Determinants of Health* (CSDH, 2008) sets out an agenda on how to tackle the various issues and inequalities outlined above. This bold document sets out a vision of change that seeks to eradicate the substantial differences in life expectancy at birth and other health inequalities within a generation. The basic premise is that no biological reasons exist to adequately explain those inequalities. Rather, the causes of inequality and poor health are to be located in social and economic structures. The report identifies that to do so requires cooperation, alliance building and participation on a global scale. The specific recommendations of the report are threefold (CSDH, 2000: 2):

1 Improve daily living conditions.
2 Tackle the inequitable distribution of power, money and resources.
3 Measure and understand the problem and assess the impact of action.

More specifically, the Report notes that increased tobacco use, obesity and car ownership also pose notable public health risks. What is notable about such 'health risks' is that they are social in origin, therefore capable of being countered on a social level through legislation, health promotion or deeper changes in how multinational companies (such as tobacco companies) are allowed to operate.

The increasing extent of globalization in the twenty-first century will prompt and create many profound changes in all aspects of people's lives. The so-called 'credit crunch' of 2008 and 2009 provides a powerful example of how globalization inextricably connects people around the world. The same interconnections exist in health with the causes, cures and means of improving health the world over bound up with the actions and decisions not of single nation-states but the coordinated activities of people and organizations across the globe.

REFERENCES AND FURTHER READING

CSDH (Commission on Social Determinants of Health) (2008) *Closing the Gap in a Generation: Health Equity through Action on the Social Determinants of Health. Final Report of the Commission on Social Determinants of Health.* Geneva: World Health Organization.

Lee, K., Buse, K. and Fustukian, S. (eds) (2002) *Health Policy in a Globalising World.* Cambridge: Cambridge University Press.

Ranson, M. K., Beaglehole, R., Correa, C. M., Mirza, Z., Buse, K. and Drager, N. (2002) 'The public health implications of multilateral trade agreements', in K. Lee, K. Buse, and S. Fustukian (eds), *Health Policy in a Globalising World*. Cambridge: Cambridge University Press.

Scriven, A. and Garman, S. (2005) *Promoting Health: Global Perspectives*. Basingstoke: Palgrave Macmillan.

Wilkinson, R. G. (2008) *Unhealthy Societies: The Afflictions of Inequality*. London: Routledge.

WHO (World Health Organisation) (2008) *The Global Burden of Disease: 2004 Update*. Geneva: World Health Organization.

C. Y.

global health

Part 4
Health Beliefs and Health Behaviour

Models of
health behaviour

A key target of research in the health domain is to improve our understanding of health behaviours (any behaviour undertaken to prevent illness/disease or to optimize health). This goal raises the following questions. What health beliefs are linked to the uptake of health screening? What factors predict which individuals will quit smoking? Who is most at risk for having unprotected sex? Investigating issues such as these can help us to predict which individuals will display unhealthy behaviours and help us to develop targeted interventions to improve health.

One approach to understanding and predicting health behaviour is to apply a model of health behaviour. Health behaviour models examine the thoughts and beliefs which predict behaviour. These models are based on the assumption that behaviour results from the individual rationally weighing up the potential pros and cons of the behaviour in question.

A few of the most commonly used models in the health field, the Health Belief Model, the Theory of Planned Behaviour, and the Stages of Change model will be discussed next.

The Health Belief Model or HBM is the one of the most widely used social cognition model. It was developed by Rosenstock (1966) then later developed by Becker and colleagues throughout the 1970s and 1980s.

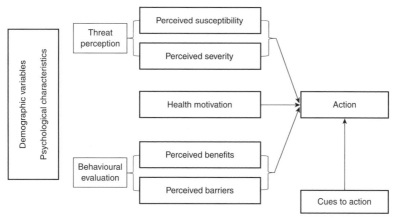

Figure 1   *Health Belief Model, Rosenstock (1966)*

The two main components of the HBM are the threat perception and behavioural evaluation aspects. The first of these, threat perception, is made up of an individual's perceived susceptibility and perceived severity. Perceived susceptibility relates to beliefs about how likely it is we will be affected by negative outcomes of the behaviour and perceived severity relates to beliefs about how serious these negative outcomes are likely to be. If we take the example of diet, the individual's threat perception would be made up of beliefs about how susceptible they are to the detrimental effects of poor diet (e.g. 'my diet could put me at risk of heart disease') and how severe the effects of this are likely to be (e.g. 'heart disease could kill me'). If the individual's threat perception results in a belief that their health may be threatened, they are likely to change their behaviour (e.g. improve their diet).

The second main component of the HBM is the behavioural evaluation process. This process involves the individual 'weighing up' of the perceived benefits and barriers of the behaviour change. Continuing with the example of healthy eating, if a person holds the belief that improving their diet will improve their body shape, this would be a benefit. Holding a number of beliefs about benefits will make it more likely that the individual will make the behaviour change. Individuals are also likely to hold beliefs about potential barriers to change (e.g. 'I don't know much about healthy eating'). If they feel, however, that the barrier can be overcome (e.g. 'I'll ask my GP for advice') or if the benefits outweigh the barriers, then the behavioural evaluation process is likely to weigh in favour of behaviour change. The HBM further suggests that behaviour is also influenced by an individual's health motivation – how much they care about their health. The HBM also predicts that 'cues to action' will influence behaviour. Cues to action can be external, such as messages in the media or advice from health professionals. They can also be internal, such as experiencing symptoms and perceiving them to be related to health (e.g. 'I'm breathless because I'm overweight').

The HBM has been applied to a wide range of behaviours and, in general, studies have supported a relationship between the components of the HBM and behaviour. A number of studies have reported, however, conflicting findings with respect to the perceived severity and perceived susceptibility components. Contradictory to the prediction of the HBM, low severity and low susceptibility (rather than high) were linked to behaviour. These studies suggest that for some health behaviours, action is sometimes more likely to occur when the illness is perceived to be less severe and/or less likely to be personally experienced. Something other than the HBM components is likely to be playing a role here, perhaps the availability of resources or the stigma of the behaviour in question.

Another theory that helps us understand behaviour is the Theory of Planned Behaviour (TPB), a model based on the earlier theory of reasoned action (Fishbein and Ajzen, 1975).

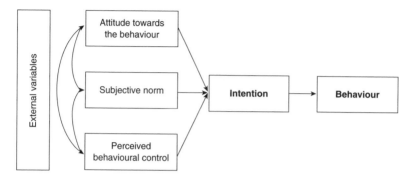

Figure 2   *Theory of Planned Behaviour, Azjen (1988)*

The model proposes that intention to engage in a behaviour is determined by an individual's attitude towards the behaviour, their perception of the subjective norm, and their perceived behavioural control (PBC). It also proposes that these components are influenced by external variables (personality traits, demographic characteristics, and environmental influences). The 'subjective norm' is a person's beliefs about what important people think they should do in relation to the behaviour. Important people in this context are figures from their social circle whose opinion or respect is valued. A person will be more likely to take up exercise, for example, if they feel that their partner wishes them to do so. An individual's perceived ability to change a particular behaviour is incorporated into the perceived behavioural control element of the model. This perceived ability to control the behaviour is also sometimes referred to as self-efficacy. The TPB predicts that a person will have a greater intention to exercise if they have a positive attitude towards exercising, if they believe that important people want them to exercise, and if they feel they have the ability to take up exercising. Greater intention is proposed by the model to link to a greater likelihood of the person engaging in the behaviour.

The TPB has received support from studies applying the model to a variety of health-related behaviours. A recent meta-analysis of 56 studies applying the TPB to a range of health behaviours reported that the model accounted for 41 per cent of the variance in individuals' intentions and

34 per cent of the variance in individuals' future behaviour (Godin and Kok, 1996). Unlike the HBM, the TPB includes a role for environmental and social influences on behaviour through the subjective norm component. Although it includes some role for past behaviour within the perceived behavioural control component (i.e. those who have performed the behaviour successfully in the past will have a greater sense of control over the behaviour), some researchers have argued that a distinct 'past behaviour' component is missing from the model.

STAGE MODELS

The Stages of Change model or Transtheoretical model (TTM; Di Clemente and Prochaska, 1982) of health behaviour is the dominant stage model used in the health field. Stage models propose that individuals progress (and regress) through a number of stages of readiness before adopting or quitting a behaviour. The stages of the model are shown in Table 1 and consist of three pre-action stages (pre-contemplation, contemplation and preparation) and two action stages (action and maintenance). The model proposes that individuals move through the stages in the order shown in Table 1. The model states that at each change of stage a decisional balance process occurs where the individual weighs up the pros and cons of changing the behaviour. The TTM also aims to explain relapse. It suggests that individuals may relapse to an earlier stage of change and may cycle through the stages several times before they have made a stable long-term change to their behaviour.

Table 1 *Stages of change*

Stage of change	Definition of stage
Precontemplation	No intention to take action in the next six months
	e.g. 'I have no desire to stop smoking'
Contemplation	Intends to take action in next six months
	e.g 'Perhaps I should think about stopping'
Preparation	Intends to take action in next month and has taken some steps towards changing
	e.g. 'I want to stop, I'm going to cut down and buy nicotine patches'
Action	Has changed behaviour for less than six months
	e.g. 'I have stopped smoking'
Maintenance	Has changed behaviour for more than six months
	e.g. 'I'm a non-smoker, I've not been smoking for seven months now'

The TTM has been widely applied to research and used as a basis for intervention work. Individuals in a particular stage can be provided with tailored interventions appropriate for the stage they are at. There are a number of criticisms of the model, however. Some researchers have questioned the helpfulness of assigning people to a category. They argue that saying a smoker is contemplative is simplistic and does not take into account their intention to change. Furthermore, categorizing people in this way may lead to them not receiving the help and support that may make them significantly improve their health. An additional criticism is that the process of transition between stages is unclear and more long-term research is needed to clarify progression and regression.

In summary, social psychological models of health behaviour are a valuable tool helping us to better understand human behaviour. They provide a testable focus for research as well as introducing avenues for intervention. The main criticism of many of these models is that although they may predict an individual's intention to behave, this does not always mean they predict actual behaviour. This issue is referred to as the 'intention–behaviour gap'. One way this gap may be addressed is through the amalgamation of model concepts. There is considerable overlap between the concepts of different models which could benefit from clarification and this has led researchers to call for the integration of the most predictive components into one model. Finally, while health behaviour models help us to explore individuals' behaviour, they do place the responsibility of health behaviour change on the individual and do not take into account the influence that the social and economic environment has on the health of individuals and communities.

REFERENCES

Ajzen, I. (1985) 'From intention to actions: a theory of planned behaviour', in J. Kuhl and J. Beckman (eds), *Action-Control: From Cognition to Behaviour*. Heidelberg: Springer, pp. 11–39.

Di Clemente, C. C. and Prochaska, J. O. (1982) 'Self-change and therapy change of smoking behaviour: a comparison of processes of change in cessation and maintenance', *Addictive Behaviours*, 7: 133–42.

Fishbein, M. and Ajzen, I. (1975) *Belief, Attitude, Intention, and Behavior*. New York: Wiley.

Godin, G. and Kok, G. (1996) 'The theory of planned behaviour: a review of its applications to health-related behaviours', *American Journal of Health Promotion*, 11: 87–98.

Rosenstock, I. M. (1966) 'Why people use health services', *Millbank Memorial Fund Quarterly*, 44: 94–124.

health behaviour models of

E. D.

EXAMPLE OBESITY

Individual behaviour has historically been considered a product of free will, but increasingly health behaviour is recognized as being constrained by an individual's social and material circumstances. There is evidence that attitudes and beliefs do exert an effect on behaviour, so that people who hold a positive set of beliefs that behaviour is strongly linked to health outcomes are more likely to adopt 'healthy' lifestyles). Nonetheless, when social class and income are controlled in health surveys, the influence of such beliefs largely disappears (Blaxter, 1990). It is now generally acknowledged that the relationship between health knowledge and health behaviour is not at all a straightforward one (see **Health promotion**).

Eating and physical activity are two critical behaviours with the potential to influence energy balance in the body. It is now widely accepted that changes in lifestyle and patterns of consumption have followed wider social, economic and cultural change within modern societies and have resulted in systematic reductions in human energy expenditure. These include changes in employment patterns that have led to a reduction in manual labour and an increase in sedentary non-manual jobs, longer working hours (which have resulted in more limited opportunities for other forms of activity during the working day), widespread car ownership, and the rise of labour-saving devices for use at home and work. Nevertheless, the impact of these changes in the physical activity of children is less clear, this is despite evidence of reductions in walking and cycling to school. For children, other factors may also be relevant, such as the increased fears of parents about unsupervised outdoor play for children.

Increasingly, being overweight is becoming the norm for adults in Britain. In 2004, 23.6 per cent of adult men and 23.8 per cent of adult women were deemed to be obese. Obesity rates have more than doubled in the past 25 years., and are estimated to rise by 2035, to 47 per cent and 36 per cent for adult men and women respectively. The current total annual cost to the NHS of overweight and obesity (i.e. the treatment of obesity and its consequences) has been estimated at £1 billion, and the total impact on employment may be as much as £10 billion (Foresight Report, 2007: 41).

Measuring dietary intake in daily life outside the laboratory remains problematic, but by combining data from different kinds of research, a number of specific dietary risk factors for obesity have been identified. These include foods with a high energy density, diets high in fat and low in fibre, and the consumption of sugar-rich drinks, the effects of which may be magnified if a person habitually consumes large portion sizes. These identified risk factors would seem to provide promising targets for health interventions to effect change in behaviours. However, in practice, the specific causes of obesity

> differ between population groups and across a person's life course, with the accumulation of excess fat, and therefore weight, being the end result of a variety of causal pathways…the multifactorial condition of obesity is inherently unsuited to a 'one size fits all' approach. (Foresight Report, 2007)

This multi-causal pathways model is illustrated in Figure 1.

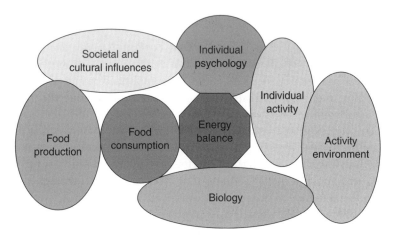

Figure 1   *Obesity system: causal pathways thematic map*

The concept of a 'family of obesities' is a useful way of recognizing the complexity of the causes of obesity within society and, as a consequence, research is increasingly turning to an examination of the social and cultural context within which these food and activity-related habits and beliefs develop (Foresight Report, 2007: 43). Some of the social and cultural contexts of obesity that have been identified would include (among many others) the following factors:

- Social pressures to consume: An increasing exposure to food advertising combined with the greater affordability of processed food.
- Increasing social acceptability of 'fatness': This development, however, is complicated by the promotion of an ideal 'slim' body image within the media.
- Changing socio-cultural valuation of food: This in part reflects the growth in working hours for both men and women with a commensurate reduction in time available for food preparation. As a consequence, less value may now be placed on family mealtimes with the result that there has been a diminishing of parental control over children's diet.
- Greater availability of 'passive entertainment': TV, computer games, internet.
- Greater urbanization with opportunities for physical activity reduced. In relation to children the lack of availability for outdoor play in many urban schools has led to a diminishing of the importance of physical sports in the curriculum.
- Greater reliance on car use and ownership for transport.

Social epidemiological studies undertaken in North America and Europe have consistently reported the existence of significant socio-economic class differences in dietary intake. Diet has been implicated as one of the key variables accounting for the overall poorer health of those in the lower socio-economic classes; within Britain people belonging to higher social classes generally have healthier diets. In terms of foods consumed, it has been found that there are also important social differences in the way in which mothers take health, costs and the taste preferences of their family into account when buying and preparing food. Middle-class mothers have been found to have as their primary consideration the 'goodness' or health value of foods, while working-class mothers tend to prioritize the cost of food and the preferences of their families over their health value (for example, Calnan, 1990; Hupkens et al., 2000). The explanation for these findings relate not only to levels of education of the mothers, but also available family income.

Rather than seeing individual health lifestyles as a distinct set of choices made between possible actions and as potentially remedial by increasing health knowledge, health behaviour can alternatively be seen as a routinized feature of everyday life guided by a practical or implicit logic. These daily practices or individual 'dispositions' (following the work of Bourdieu, 1984) are formed in different ways reflecting an individual's particular social position and their socialization into an associated set of 'worldviews' (described by Bourdieu as an individual's 'habitus'). Thus, in a very practical way, food choices can be conceived of as being a social attribute of an individual reflecting shared social attitudes and cultural conventions. Bourdieu conceptualizes these choices as reflecting individual 'taste' (referring to consumption behaviour and of lifestyle preferences rather than the physical sensation of tasting). Important social class differences in 'taste' or preferences have been found to exist in relation to dietary intake as well as the manner in which food is consumed. These social differences can be seen as manifested in terms of a preference for heavy filling fatty foods seen as sustaining the body, versus health-giving, light and non-fattening foods; and also in terms of having regular family meals around the table versus the acceptability of irregular 'grazing' of food in front of the television.

REFERENCES AND FURTHER READING

Blaxter, M. (1990) *Health and Lifestyles*. London: Routledge.

Bourdieu, P. (1984) *Distinction: A Social Critique of the Judgement of Taste*. London: Routledge.

Calnan, M. (1990) 'Food and health: a comparison of beliefs and practices in middle and working class households', in S. Cunningham-Burley (ed.), *Readings in Medical Sociology*, London: Routledge, pp. 9–36.

Denny-Wilson, E. and Campbell, K. (2008) 'Eating behaviour and obesity: Editorial', *British Medical Journal*, 337: 1926.

Foresight Report (2007) *Tackling Obesities: Future Choices*. London: Government Office for Science.

Hupkens, C., Knibbe, R. and Drop, M. (2000) 'Social Class differences in food consumption', *European Journal of Public Health*, 10(2): 108–13.

Murcott, A. (2002) 'Nutrition and inequalities', *European Journal of Public Health*, 12(3): 203–7.

I. C.

healthy lifestyle and consumption patterns

Lay knowledge and illness attribution

An understanding of health and illness is not purely the privileged knowledge of the medical profession, many sophisticated, complex but different understandings of health are also held by ordinary people; and this knowledge is termed 'lay'. These lay understandings of health and illness are informed by a complex array of cultural, gendered, class-based and generational traditions and norms, in addition to personal and familial experiences (see **The social model of health**). Lay knowledge serves to inform, mediate and modulate experiences, interpretations and responses to illness.

Too often in the past, lay knowledge of health has been dismissed (by professionals and policy-makers) as being little more than a set of ill-informed subjective beliefs lacking in rigour. Yet understanding how people both construct and interpret the health of others and themselves by establishing a mutually reciprocal dialogue between professional and lay person is vital for any successful health intervention to occur. There are serious issues, however, in claiming a direct equivalence of lay with medical knowledge and problems can arise, as Prior (2003: 45) has noted, lay people can be 'plain wrong about the causes, course and management of common forms of disease and illness'.

Blaxter (1990) has produced one of the most influential pieces of sociological research examining lay-health knowledge, citing class, age and gender as important factors in shaping understandings of health. For example, for young men, physical fitness and being able to be 'sporty' were found to be considered key attributes of strength, which contrasted with young women's more holistic interpretations that emphasized feeling good with ideas about being able to cope with life as being important. For older people, being able to 'get about' was important, but health for them was contextual. One could feel healthy while having an on-going disability or infirmity (see **Functionality**).

Turning to psychological perspectives, we find much shared ground with the sociological understanding of how individuals make sense of becoming ill. For psychologists, individuals experiencing illness will often explain their illness by attributing to it a specific cause. For example, an individual who catches a cold may attribute this to being run down. Similarly someone who gets a migraine may feel this is due to stress. Attribution theorists argue that this inherent human nature to explain events is due to how we see the world. Attribution theory (Heider, 1958) states that we have a tendency to view our social world as being predictable and controllable. Theorists argue that the process of attribution occurs along a number of dimensions as follows:

- *Internality vs. externality*: e.g., 'My failure to pass my driving test is because of my poor performance' versus 'My failure is due to the examiner's unfair treatment'.
- *Stability vs. instability*: e.g., 'I will never be able pass my driving test' versus 'I can pass if I take it again'.
- *Non-specificity vs. specificity*: e.g., 'My failure to pass is reflective of my overall poor ability' versus 'My failure to pass is only specific to this one driving test'.
- *Controllability vs. uncontrollability*: e.g., 'The cause of my failure to pass was down to me' versus 'My failure was not under my control'.

Attribution theory has been successfully applied to understanding illness and health behaviour. Illness-related attributions have been shown to vary across culture and time. In the Middle Ages, people were likely to attribute illness and disease to evil spirits. Treatment was therefore likely to involve a priest and often included torturing the body to drive out the evil spirit. Illness was also seen as God's punishment for doing evil things. In modern western culture these beliefs are much less prevalent. The most commonly held illness attributions in western cultures follow biomedical and bio-psychosocial models of illness. In these models health and illness are related to the physical body but with psychological and sociological influences on health acknowledged. Illness is seen as person-centred and attributed to natural causes such as infection, stress, organic deterioration, accident or violence. Management of the illness reflects this natural attribution and is typically undertaken by an expert trained in diagnosis and treatment.

In other cultures throughout the world, different illness attributions exist. In Chinese medicine, illness and treatment focus on a balance between the elements and energy. Ayurvedic medicine in India and Nepal attributes health to the flow of substances through various channels in the body. Other cultures may also apply a supernatural causation to illness. Three general types of supernatural causation appear to exist.

The first type, *mystical causation*, is where illness is seen as a consequence of the victim's behaviour. For example, the illness is caused by astrological influences, contact with a polluting object or person, or mystical retribution due to a violation of taboos or morals. The second type of supernatural illness attribution is *animistic causation*, where illness is caused by the behaviour of God or a supernatural entity like a soul or ghost. The final type of supernatural illness attribution is *magical causation* where the illness is caused as a deliberate act by another human being using magical means. Magical causation includes sorcery (where a human uses magical techniques) and witchcraft (where a human has magical powers). Research examining the prevalence of supernatural illness attributions worldwide found that more illnesses were perceived to be supernatural rather than natural in origin.

Whether natural or supernatural, a person's illness attributions are likely to impact on their health behaviour. For example, if a person with diabetes attributes their illness to an external cause, rather than due to their own behaviour, they may be less likely to follow a healthy eating plan. The controllability dimension of illness attributions has also been linked to behaviour. For example, an individual with hypertension will be more likely to attend appointments if they believe the illness to be controllable rather than if they feel it is outwit their control. A great deal of research has examined this controllability dimension of illness attribution using the concept of health locus of control. The multidimensional health locus of control questionnaire (Wallston et al., 1978) evaluates whether an individual attributes an internal or external locus of control with regard to their health. An internal health locus of control indicates the person believes themselves to be responsible for their health. An external locus of control indicates that the person believes other influences determine their health. These influences can be either powerful others (e.g. doctors or health professionals) or fate/luck. Research in this area has found that health locus of control is related to behaviour change (e.g. quitting smoking), and the type of communication style they need from their health professional.

Evident in this account of lay knowledge are the complexity and subtlety that exist in ordinary people's sense-making in relation to health and disease. People should always be understood as active agents in how they make sense of their lives and being healthy or ill.

REFERENCES AND FURTHER READING

Heider, F. (1958)*The Psychology of Interpersonal Relations*. New York: John Wiley and Sons. Cited in M. Hewstone, F. D. Finchman and J. Foster (eds) (2005) *Psychology*. Oxford: The British Psychological Society and Blackwell Publishing.

Prior, L. (2003) 'Belief, knowledge and expertise: the emergence of the lay expert in medical sociology', *Sociology of Health and Illness*, 25(3): 41–57.

Wallston, K. A., Wallston, B. S. and DeVillis, R. (1978) 'Development of the Multi-dimensional Health Locus of Control (MHLC) scales', *Health Education Monographs*, 6: 161–70.

C. Y. /E. D.

Personality and health

What makes one person develop disease while another remains healthy? Is there a link between a person's personality and how healthy they are?

The links between personality and health have been explored for many years. The ancient Greeks believed that both health and personality could be linked to an individual's balance of the four bodily humors: black bile, yellow bile, phlegm and blood. It was believed that if a person developed an excess of one of the four humors then both personality and health would be affected. For example, if an individual developed an excess of black bile, this would lead to melancholy and depression as well as diseases such as cancer, while an excess of phlegm led to a sluggish, unemotional personality and diseases such as rheumatism. More recently, in the 1950s, a great deal of interest was paid to the proposal of a Type A personality and its impact upon health. An individual with a Type A personality was defined as someone who is always in a hurry, competitive and readily becomes hostile. In contrast a person who did not display these characteristics was called Type B. Years of research into the link between Type A personality and health produced mixed results. Researchers conclude that high levels of competitiveness and hostility do, in some circumstances, increase the risk of coronary heart disease. However, being hurried generally does not appear to be a risk factor (Friedman, 2007). Following on from Type A research, further personality types have also been proposed. Type C personality is proposed to be prone to developing cancer and is characterized by repression, hopelessness and apathy. Type D personalities have high levels of negative emotions coupled with a greater tendency to inhibit expression of emotions and are hypothesized to be at greater risk of cardiac events.

A more comprehensive approach to studying the influence of personality on health is to investigate individual traits; characteristics of individuals that are similar over a range of situations. Many researchers believe that the traits that make up personality can be divided up into five major dimensions known as the 'Big Five' (Goldberg, 1981). These dimensions are described in Table 1.

Research has investigated the link between these five dimensions of personality and health outcome. Friedman and colleagues (1995a, 1995b) investigated the association between conscientiousness and longevity. Children were measured for conscientiousness aged 11 through parent and teacher ratings and followed over seven decades. Adults who were conscientious as children were shown to live significantly longer than their more careless peers. The possible reasons for this finding include a link between conscientiousness and behaviour. Conscientious people were less likely to smoke and drink heavily and more likely to engage in health-promoting behaviours such as exercise and healthy eating. They were also less likely to die from violence which the researchers suggest may highlight an avoidance of risk in conscientious individuals.

There is a widespread belief that agreeable, cheerful, happy people will have better health and there is research to support this notion. However, studies do not always support this common-sense view. Some research suggests that cheerful/optimistic people die earlier than those who are less cheerful (Friedman et al., 1993). Friedman and colleagues followed children into adulthood and compared those rated by parents and teachers as cheerful and optimistic. The cheerful children actually died earlier in adulthood than those rated as less cheerful. Although this may seem to go against what we might predict, follow-up research suggested that the cheerful children grew up to be more likely to take risks, and also drank and smoked more than the less cheerful comparison

Table 1 *The Big Five*

Dimension of the Big Five	Description
Openness	How ready an individual is to experience the unfamiliar. Individuals scoring low on openness are conformist, unreflective and direct, while individuals high on this dimension are imaginative, reflective and unconventional.
Conscientiousness	Degree to which an individual is organized, thorough and motivated to achieve goals. Individuals low on conscientiousness are careless and undependable. High conscientiousness scorers are dependable, scrupulous and fussy.
Extraversion	How sociable, talkative and assertive an individual is. Extraversion is the opposite of introversion. Extraverts are individuals who are talkative, adventurous and impulsive while introverts are shy, reserved and unadventurous.
Agreeableness	How concerned an individual is with maintaining social harmony. High scores on the agreeableness scale reflect a desire to get on with others and are associated with greater empathy, consideration and helpfulness. Low scorers are likely to be less concerned with others' welfare and are more likely to be unhelpful, inconsiderate, suspicious and unfriendly.
Neuroticism	Degree of emotional stability. Individuals scoring high on the neuroticism dimension are likely to be nervous, insecure and worrying. Low neuroticism is linked to a calm, composed and relaxed demeanour.

group. One suggestion to explain the difference in findings is that the individual's appraisals of the situation is key. If an individual's health is affected and they are required to adhere to a difficult treatment regime, cheerfulness could impact upon this in two ways. It may make the individual more accepting of the situation and their good humour and coping skills may make them more likely to stick with the treatment. Cheerfulness in this situation, however, could also be potentially detrimental to their health. The individual may believe that 'everything will work out fine for me anyway'. This underlying optimistic viewpoint may actually make them less likely to follow a difficult treatment plan as they feel so optimistic that they have little motivation to do so.

Studies in the 1980s examined whether a pessimistic disposition made individuals more likely to experience health complications. Peterson and colleagues (1988) examined data from students taken in 1946 and examined long-term health outcomes of the students at age 55. Peterson found that a pessimistic personality type (with the belief that bad events occur because of stable, global and internal factors) predicted death or poor health at age 55. Why should it be that pessimists are likely to face poorer health? A number of possible mechanisms exist. Perhaps when faced with illness, pessimists are more likely to become passive and fail to seek medical advice thinking that any medical advice would be 'a waste of time'. Furthermore, pessimists may be less likely to have a strong social support system, resulting in poorer coping skills. Further research (Kubzansky et al., 2001) suggests that an optimistic personality style is protective against coronary heart disease in older men.

Neuroticism has also been linked to poorer health but the association is far from clear. People who are neurotic tend to be anxious, tense and prone to depression and stress. A great deal of research links diseases with higher levels of anxiety and depression but the reasons why this is the case are uncertain. For example, Frasure-Smith and colleagues (1993) found that after a heart attack, patients who were depressed were significantly more likely to die than those who were not depressed. What we cannot tell, however, is whether the depression faced by patients causes poorer health or is in fact itself caused by poorer health. Moreover, in some cases a degree of neuroticism may actually be beneficial to health. Neurotic people are likely to be more aware of bodily symptoms and, for that reason, may be more likely to identify illness and disease at an earlier stage and seek treatment earlier than their non-neurotic counterparts. There is some evidence to back this up, Brickman et al. (1996) found that renal patients with moderate levels of neuroticism fared better than those with low or high neuroticism. Therefore, a degree of neuroticism may actually benefit health.

THEORIES OF PERSONALITY–HEALTH LINK

A variety of potential mechanisms exist to explain the personality–health link. Personality determines how individuals respond to their environment. Personality may influence how likely it is that an individual will experience stress, and determine their emotional, behavioural and physiological responses to stress. This psychophysiological link between personality and stress can explain some of the individual differences seen in health outcomes (see **Stress and coping**). Individual differences in personality may explain differences in the availability of social support and therefore impact upon health through differences in individuals' ability to cope with illness. For example, certain personality traits may make it more likely that a person will have a large group of people around them able to offer emotional support. Those individuals with greater emotional support are likely to cope better when experiencing ill health. A further explanation of the personality–health link is that personality determines health behaviours. For instance, an impulsive person may be more likely to take up smoking, thereby having a detrimental effect on their long-term health. Personality will therefore have an indirect impact upon health through people's choices regarding health behaviours. A further point to consider is the question of cause and effect. Is it really the case that personality variables change health or is it that aspects of the illness itself result in changes to an individual's personality? Perhaps aspects of the illness experience (e.g. the unemployment experienced as a result or the reactions/behaviour of others) may produce a change in an individual's personality. A previously cheerful and optimistic person may change when faced with illness. A long spell unable to work coupled with the negative reactions of friends and colleagues may result in the individual becoming pessimistic and more guarded than before. A substantial number of studies in this area cannot answer this question as they apply a cross-sectional design. This means that they look at health and personality at one point in time rather than applying a longitudinal design which follows individuals over a number of years. Cross-sectional research cannot shed light on the question of cause and effect with respect to personality and health, therefore further long-term longitudinal studies are necessary.

REFERENCES

Brickman, A. L., Yount, S. E., Blaney, N. T., Rothberg, S. T. and De-Nour, A. K. (1996) 'Personality traits and long-term health status: the influence of neuroticism and conscientiousness on renal deterioration in Type-1 diabetes', *Psychosomatics: Journal of Consultation Liaison Psychiatry*, 37: 459–68. Cited in H. S. Friedman, *Foundations of Health Psychology*. Oxford: Oxford University Press, pp. 172–99.

Frasure-Smith, N., Lesperance, F. and Talajic, M. (1993) 'Depression following myocardial infarction: impact on 6-month survival', *Journal of American Medical Association*, 70(15): 1819–25.

personality and health

Friedman, H. S. (2007) 'Personality, disease, and self-healing', in H. S. Friedman, *Foundations of Health Psychology*. Oxford: Oxford University Press, pp. 172–99.

Friedman, H. S., Tucker, J., Tomlinson-Keasey, C., Schwartz, J., Wingard, D. and Criqui, M. H. (1993) 'Does childhood personality predict longevity?', *Journal of Personality and Social Psychology*, 65: 176–85.

Friedman, H. S., Tucker, J., Schwartz, J. E., Martin, L. R., Tomilnson-Keasey, C., Wingard, D., et al. (1995a) 'Childhood conscientiousness and longevity: health behaviours and cause of death', *Journal of Personality and Social Psychology*, 68: 696–703.

Friedman, H. S., Tucker, J. S., Schwartz, J. E., Tomlinson-Keasey, C., Martin, L. R., Wingard, D. L., et al. (1995b) 'Psychosocial predictors of longevity: the ageing and death of the "Termites"', *American Psychologist*, 50: 69–78.

Goldberg, L. (1981) 'Language and individual differences: the search for universals in personality lexicons', in L. Wheeler, *Review of Personality and Social Psychology*. Beverly Hills, CA: Sage, pp. 141–65.

Kubzansky, L. D., Sparrow, D., Vokonas, P. and Kawachi, I. (2001) 'Is the glass half empty or half full? A prospective study of optimism and coronary heart disease in the normative aging study', *Psychosomatic Medicine*, 63: 910–16.

Peterson, C., Siegelman, M. E. and Valliant, G. E. (1988) 'Pessimistic explanatory style is a risk factor for physical illness: a thirty-five-year longitudinal study', *Journal of Personality and Social Psychology*, 55(1): 23–7.

E. D.

key concepts in
health studies

Embodiment

The concept of embodiment perceives human existence as the interweaving of mind, body and society. The body is not just a biological entity but is conceived as fully being part of the human sense of self and an important element in individual and social identity.

The body has until recently been 'off-limits' to the social sciences as an area to study and theorize. It is the natural sciences that are commonly accepted as being the only disciplines that can advance any understanding of the human body. In courses that concern health, meditations on the body have been traditionally left to biology and anatomy lessons. Here a particular perspective of the body is presented as being a complex, but ultimately mechanical, entity consisting of related series of systems and processes. There has been a proliferation of writing and research in recent years concerning the human body within sociology, psychology and the wider social sciences (for example, Williams and Bendelow, 1998; Williams, 2003; Turner, 2008). Such non-medical material on the human body has explored many different aspects of the body in a variety of sub-cultural and mainstream cultural practices. What is interestingly demonstrated by the social science material is that the study of the human body can be much more than the 'blood-and -bones' approach of the natural sciences. The body should rather be seen as also belonging to the social and psychological, and an important element in the complexities of being human that stresses how we are in the world, how we create and project our identities and how our bodies are shaped by society and how at times the human body can shape society. It is to these concerns that the concept of embodiment speaks. At its most basic, embodiment understands that human existence is the interweaving of the mind, the body and society.

Many reasons exist why embodiment is important for Health Studies. The main reason is that embodiment offers a much more rounded and holistic understanding of the body that assists us in understanding how people experience health and illness. There are other reasons too and these are outlined and explored in this entry.

It is useful first of all to consider some of the philosophical aspects of embodiment. For a start, to be an active human being who functions within a wider society, creates cultures, perceives other people and makes cognitive sense of reality, entails that we have to accept that this is done with and through our physical, and biological bodies. In short, without the body we would not exist at all! However, this does not say that everything can be reduced to biology, as embodiment is about what we purposefully do and experience with our bodies and how that is mediated by the societies and cultures in which we exist.

Interest in the body has also been prompted by a variety of trends and impulses inherent within contemporary society. Many of these are connected with how we live our lives and the challenges and issues we face as a society and as individuals in this particular phase of modernity. According to Giddens (1991), the body has gained importance in an increasingly changing and fluid world as one of relatively few fixed reference points for our sense of self, over which we can potentially exert control. The traditions and social structures such as religion, social class and geographical place that identities were formally embedded in are being swept aside in a mobile and rapidly transforming global society. In the past, self-identity was, in some ways, easier to maintain.

embodiment

Identity was, in effect, 'off-the-peg', already made for you according to your location in society. That is not currently the case and in this constantly altering phase of modernity, people have to look to the one resource that is constant, their body, as a source and resource of identity. So, instead of drawing our identity from, say, occupation, one has to construct and reconstruct one's self-identity using one's body.

Using the body as a source of identity is further heightened in a consumer society. Consumerism, in addition to the purchase of goods and services, also carries a strong 'moral' dimension, with status being accorded to individuals on their ability to manipulate and articulate consumerist symbols (see **Health care consumerism and patient choice**).

We can all bear witness to how this process is enacted in daily life. Buying the 'right' fashionable clothes is one strategy, but the body inside must also be of certain dimensions; toned, sleek and without any 'unsightly' fat. The worth of an individual is rightly or wrongly based upon their articulation of consumerist norms: a moral dimension to the body. When the body does not accord to those norms a person can experience a range of negative emotions. The association between consumer culture, poor body image, and eating disorders has been noted by the British Medical Association (2000).

Chronic illness and the implications that long-term, often degenerative disease has for people, provide another prompt for interest in embodiment. For many people, ill health, especially the chronic illnesses, can often have a highly damaging effect on the body. As cells mutate and form cancers or various elements of neurological systems misfire, causing limbs to move in ways that other people may find unsettling, another consequence of ill health's disturbances on the body becomes apparent. Given that the body is the medium through which personal identity is lived and presented, change brought about by a chronic illness and disability will potentially lead to a destabilization of that identity (see **Biographical disruption**). The notion of a relationship between biography, embodiment and health can also be found in understanding older people's health. Much research has indicated that it is not simply a function of being old that affects the health of older people. One should instead focus on how a lifetime's experiences throughout the life course influence older people's health in all sort of subtle and quite direct ways. In effect, life events-experiences are 'recorded' onto the body. If those experiences and events were of a hard life framed by poverty, then the story they will tell in older years could be one of ill-health and disability. Blane et al. usefully summarize this point:

The body can be seen as a mechanism which stores the past benefits and dis-benefits to which it has been exposed, either because damage at a critical period of development causes irreparable loss or because the effects of various types of damage accumulate over time. (2004: 2171)

Overall, the concept of embodiment provides a creative and holistic approach to understanding the human body, beyond the traditional reductionist approach found in the natural sciences.

REFERENCES AND FURTHER READING

Blane, D., Higgs, P., Hyde, M. and Wiggins, R. (2004) 'Life course influences on quality of life in early old age', *Social Science and Medicine*, 58: 2171–9.
British Medical Association (2000) *Eating Disorders, Body Image and the Media*. London: BMJ Books.
Giddens, A. (1991) *Modernity and Self-Identity*. London: Polity.
Turner, B. (2008) *The Body and Society*, 3rd edn. London: Sage.
Williams, S. J. (2003) *Medicine and the Body*. London: Sage.
Williams, S. J. and Bendelow, G. (1998) *The Lived Body: Sociological Themes, Embodied Issues*. London: Routledge.

C. Y.

Stress and coping

WHAT IS STRESS?

Stress is a difficult concept to define. Different people are likely to have differing explanations of what stress feels like to them. Furthermore, researchers may define the concept differently from lay people. The definition of stress as the negative emotional experience and tension that arise when an individual is faced with a stressor and he or she feels unable to cope is perhaps the most commonly used today. It is based on transactional models of stress which consider stress as an appraisal process. Under this framework, stress is the imbalance between the perceived demand of the situation and the individual's perceived ability to meet this demand. An alternative view of stress argues that individuals have a fixed tolerance level for stress. When stress becomes too great, this tolerance level is exceeded and results in physical and psychological consequences (e.g. tiredness, anxiety and muscle tension). One of the earliest models of stress is the 'flight or fight' model (Cannon, 1932). This model views stress as a physiological response to an external stressor and proposes that when we encounter a stressful situation, our body responds by releasing chemicals such as adrenaline. This reaction results in acceleration of our heart rate and breathing rate, and increased blood flow to our muscles. These physiological changes are in preparation for us to make a response either to engage in fighting the stressor or to engage in flight and attempt to escape the stressor.

If we are walking down a street, for example, and suddenly are confronted with a large angry dog, our body automatically prepares us by releasing chemicals to ready our body in order to protect ourselves. This physiological response prepares us to either physically protect ourselves from the dog or to run away and attempt escape. Although this model is supported with biological and animal research, it does not adequately explain psychological stress. More recent models of stress changed the focus from the physiological impact of stress to psychological influences and responses. These transactional models of stress view stress as a complex psychological state arising from the individual's appraisal of the situation and their own coping abilities as discussed above.

DOES STRESS IMPACT UPON HEALTH?

It is a commonly held belief that stress has a negative impact on health. Research in this area has found conflicting results making conclusions difficult. The conflicting results are likely to be due to methodological issues. Studies investigating the influence of stress on health are extremely difficult to carry out. How do we define who is stressed? Do we ask people to self-report their stress levels or try and use some kind of objective measure to rate how stressful their life is? Good quality research often requires a control group so that we can compare a 'stress-exposed' group to a 'non-stress-exposed group' but finding such a group outwith the laboratory is likely to be impossible. Research involving experimentally induced stress has, furthermore, obvious ethical problems.

Despite these difficulties, evidence suggests that stress can impact upon health and well-being. With regard to well-being, people who experience chronic stress are more likely to experience depression and anxiety. The mechanisms underlying the link with physical health are both behavioural and physiological. Research has shown that stress leads to behavioural change, resulting in an inhibition of some protective health behaviours (like exercise, eating well and sleep) along with a promotion of negative health behaviours (like smoking, alcohol and drug use). Stress can also impact upon health through physiological pathways. Recent research in the field of psychoneuroimmunology suggests that stress can influence the immune system via the nervous system (see **Work and health**). Further evidence suggests wound healing is slower in stressed participants than in non-stressed controls. Marucha et al. (1998) experimentally inflicted wounds on students at two time points: prior to major examinations and at the end of the summer holidays. The students' wounds took 40 per cent longer to heal in the high stress condition just prior to their exams. Although this was a small-scale study, it suggests that even transient exam-related stress can have consequences for health. Further evidence of a physiological mechanism underlying the stress–illness link comes from studies of chronic illnesses, like diabetes. A further physiological consequence of stress is that our blood glucose levels become raised. This elevation is particularly troublesome for individuals with diabetes who aim to keep their blood sugar at a lower level. If the individual's blood glucose remains significantly higher than desirable for an extended period of time, long-term health is likely to be affected.

Although the evidence discussed supports a relationship between stress and ill health, this relationship is not simple. It is likely that the relationship is moderated (affected) by a number of psychosocial variables such as social support, personality (see **Personality and health**) and coping. The influence of coping on stress and illness will be discussed next.

STRESS AND COPING

Coping is the individual's behavioural and cognitive efforts to manage environmental and psychological demands. In the context of stress, coping is the person's efforts to deal with stressors in an attempt to return to their normal non-stressed state. There is a debate in the coping literature as to whether coping is a personality trait or whether it is a behaviour strategy specific to a particular situation and time point. In support of the former, Roth and Cohen (1986) argue that individual differences in coping can be summarized into two opposing styles: approach coping and avoidance coping. An 'approacher' is proposed to deal with a stressor by confronting the problem through gaining information and direct action. In contrast, the 'avoider' is proposed to deal with a stressor through denial and reducing the importance of the problem. Roth and Cohen argue that there are costs and benefits related to both approaches. Avoidance prevents the individual from becoming over-whelmed, reduces initial distress and allows for gradual recognition of the threat. Delaying action, however, can be costly and avoidance may lead to a delayed psychological response to the threat. Approach allows for quick action which may mean the problem is quickly solved. A further benefit of approach is that any emotional response is expressed at the appropriate time which leads to advantages (e.g. increased support from others). The costs of approach, however, include the possibility of increased worry and distress if the situation is not changeable.

Researchers who define coping as a behavioural strategy (rather than a trait like Roth and Cohen) focus on two different coping strategies: emotion-focused and problem-focused coping. Both emotion-focused and problem-focused coping strategies can be utilized by the one person at the same time. Emotion-focused coping involves behavioural and cognitive attempts by the individual to deal with the emotional conse-quences of stress. Behavioural strategies may include distraction tech-niques such as visiting a friend, or reading a book, or may involve drinking alcohol or taking drugs. Cognitive strategies employed during emotion-focused coping can consist of denial, thinking positively and wishful thinking. When an individual applies problem-focused coping, they take action to try and manage the problem that is causing stress. They may try to reduce the demands of the stressor itself, by delegating work to colleagues or extending a deadline, or they may try and increase their resources to deal with the stressor, by making and sticking to a plan or by organizing a study group. As described, coping strategies may be adaptive and helpful to the individual or may be maladaptive (e.g. drinking more alcohol or taking drugs). A key aim of stress management work is to increase adaptive coping and reduce maladaptive coping.

STRESS MANAGEMENT

Stress management can take a variety of forms, from education about stress identification and management to psychological treatment and rehabilitation. Murphy (1996) conducted a review examining which stress management techniques were commonly used in workplace settings and investigated how effective they were. Progressive muscle relaxation (PMR) was one of the most frequently used techniques and involves the systematic tension and relaxation of muscles in the body.

Typically, the progression of tensing and relaxing starts at the feet and moves up the body. The idea behind the technique is that through repeated practice, individuals begin to learn how to identify and respond to natural muscle tension that accompanies stress. Another commonly used technique was cognitive behavioural skills training. Cognitive behavioural skills training for stress management typically involves aspects such as assertiveness training and cognitive restructuring (correcting 'faulty' thinking). A further technique was meditation which tends to entail training in developing a deeper state of relaxation or awareness. The least commonly used technique was biofeedback. This involves using a machine that translates tension in the muscles into visual or audio signals. For example, the biofeedback machine may beep rapidly when muscles are tense and slow as the individual relaxes the muscles. It is proposed to work in a similar way to PMR through helping individuals to learn to identify and respond to muscle tension. Murphy found that the most consistent and effective technique to reduce stress was meditation and the least effective was biofeedback. The greatest benefit to individuals occurred when a combination of techniques were given.

The evidence of the impact of stress on health has resulted in a greater understanding of the importance for stress reduction provision to improve the nation's health. Furthermore, recent legislation in the UK has now made it an employer's responsibility to assess their workforce for elevated stress and to introduce stress management if appropriate. Research examining the effectiveness of stress reduction training indicates that techniques such as meditation may prove useful in reducing the detrimental effects of health on health and well-being.

REFERENCES

Cannon, W. B. (1932) *The Wisdom of the Body*. New York: Norton.

Marucha, P. T., Kiecolt, J. K. and Favagehi, M. (1998) 'Mucosal wound healing is impaired by examination stress', *Psychosomatic Medicine*, 60(3): 362–5.

Murphy, L. R. (1996) 'Stress management in work settings: a critical review of the health effects', *American Journal of Health Promotion*, 11(2): 112–35.

Ross, R. (1999) 'Atherosclerosis – an inflammatory disease', *The New England Journal of Medicine*, 340: 115–26.

Roth, S. and Cohen, L. J. (1986) 'Approach, avoidance, and coping with stress', *American Psychologist*, 41(7): 813–19.

stress and coping

E. D.

Motivational interviewing in health care

Motivational interviewing (MI) has been defined as 'a directive client-centred counselling style for eliciting behaviour change by helping clients to explore and resolve ambivalence' (Rollnick and Miller, 1995). The focus of MI is helping patients talk about and resolve their ambivalence to behaviour change using their motivation, energy and commitment to do so.

Often when patients are advised by health professionals to make changes to their behaviours (like stopping smoking, or cutting down their alcohol intake), they struggle to do so. Health behaviours are likely to have been built up over a number of years and are therefore likely to include a great deal of habit and unconscious behaviour. Motivational interviewing (MI) is a technique used by a variety of health professions (e.g. nursing, medical, physiotherapy, dentistry). It was first described by Miller (1983) as an intervention for problem drinking but has since been applied to a variety of health behaviours including smoking cessation, drug addiction, and safe sex behaviour. The main aim of MI is to direct clients to explore their ambivalence to making changes and to help them to resolve this ambivalence. MI is conducted within a collaborative setting that acknowledges patient autonomy, utilizing a client-centred or patient-centred approach (see **Professional–client communication**). Therefore, shared decision making exists and the patient's right to choose and be responsible for their own health is recognized. Clients are educated about the variety of therapeutic options available to them but it is up to the individual client to choose which options they feel will be most useful to them. Just as counsellors emphasize freedom of choice, MI emphasizes that clients are responsible for their own progress.

Rollnick and Miller (1995) discuss key features of the approach that are central to MI (summarized in Table 1).

Many people working in a health setting have chosen their career due to a desire to help people. Due to this inherent drive to help people, the

Table 1 *Key features of motivational interviewing*

1. Motivation to change comes from the client, it is not imposed upon them.	MI involves aiding the client to identify their own goals and values to promote behaviour change.
2. Expressing and resolving ambivalence is the responsibility of the client rather than the counsellor.	The counsellor is there to guide the client, but it is the client who holds the key both to why change has not happened and what strategies could help facilitate change.
3. Persuasion should not be used to attempt and change behaviour.	Direct persuasion from the counsellor generally has the opposite effect from what was desired and actually increases the resistance of the client.
4. Counsellor should adopt a quiet and eliciting approach.	Persuasion, argumentation and aggressive confrontation should not be used. Pushing a client before they are ready to make a change is counter-productive.
5. A client's readiness to change behaviour fluctuates in response to the client–counsellor relationship.	If a client displays resistance or denial, this is often a sign that the counsellor has assumed a greater readiness to change than exists.
6. MI should involve a partnership not adopt expert/patient roles.	MI encourages client autonomy and freedom of choice.

urge to correct another's behaviour can become reflexive. When conducting MI it is necessary to resist this automatic response (termed by Rollnick and Miller as 'the righting reflex') because often it can have the opposite effect to what was desired because of an individual's tendency to resist persuasion. A principal goal of MI is resisting the righting reflex and instead getting the patient to voice the benefits of change themselves. The relationship between client and counsellor is extremely important to MI. The relationship should be collaborative and friendly where change is reinforced by genuine positive reinforcement (i.e. praise). The counsellor aims to increase clients' self-efficacy, i.e. their belief that they can make real changes to the target behaviour. One way this is achieved is through the collaborative partnership-style of MI. Patients with a greater sense of power, both in their relationships with health professionals and over their own health, have been shown to have better outcomes. It is important for health professionals to recognize the knowledge and expertise that patients bring to the consultation.

Traditionally the health professional was seen as having the answers and the patient the questions. However, in particular for behaviour change, it is the patient who has the greater knowledge about their lifestyle and their motivation. The principal goal of MI is, therefore, for the health professional to demonstrate empathic listening (i.e. demonstrating a caring attitude and ensuring they understand). Taking time to ensure accurate and thorough understanding is vital for success as a patient's reasons for change are highly individual and determined by a variety of inter-personal and situational factors. When conducting MI, it is important to get to the root of which factors are going to motivate a particular individual in order to make a change to their behaviour and to lead the patient to verbalize these factors for themselves. Understanding the underlying issues is also important in order for the counsellor to demonstrate empathy. Empathy involves 'seeing the world through the client's eyes' and sharing their experiences in an understanding way. When empathy is demonstrated effectively by the counsellor, the client is more able to openly discuss their experiences and is also more open to gentle challenges by the counsellor.

MI IN PRACTICE

MI counsellors use a number of interaction techniques to aid their work with clients including open-ended questions, affirmations, reflective listening and summaries. Open-ended questions are those which cannot be answered with a short answer like 'yes' or 'no'. For example, the MI counsellor may begin the first session with a client by asking an open-ended question like 'What brought you here today?'. Open-ended questions are essential in developing a client-centred approach. Traditional expert–patient relationships typically include a lot of closed questions and consequently the discussion revolves around what the 'expert' deems to be relevant, rather than what the client wishes to discuss. An MI counsellor will also use affirmations, positive reinforcement of the client's strengths, to aid behaviour change. Using affirmations may help to build a collaborative and friendly relationship with the client, however, any praise must be genuine or it may serve to damage rather than build rapport. A further interaction technique is to employ reflective listening. Reflective listening is a technique which involves listening carefully to the client and ensuring that the counsellor conducts more listening than talking. The technique also involves reflecting back what the client has just said in order to ensure both correct understanding but also to demonstrate empathy. It has been suggested that the counsellor should include three reflections for every question they ask. A final technique applied by MI counsellors is to give frequent summaries of what the client has been saying. Summaries are a way of demonstrating understanding and empathy but also a useful tool with which to highlight important points of discussion and a way to shift the client's attention to another area. When summarizing in this way, MI counsellors will tend to include an invitation for the client to correct the summary or to add anything they might have missed out, further developing a collaborative approach. A number of typical activities included in MI sessions are included in Table 2.

Table 2 *MI counselling strategies*

Reviewing a typical day

Looking back to before the behaviour started

Benefits and costs of the behaviour

Discussing stages of behaviour change in the context of the transtheoretical model (see **Models of health behaviour**)

Discussing the client's ideal self

Looking at what life would be like if behaviour continued and if it changed

Action planning for the future

EFFICACY

A number of reviews of MI interventions have been carried out. The results of these have been somewhat mixed. Hettema et al. (2005) found that while MI interventions were useful for changing some addictive behaviours, such as diet and exercise, they did not appear to be effective for smoking cessation. A further review (Grenard et al., 2006) reported that of the nine studies reviewed, five studies showed significant reductions in substance use in MI intervention groups compared to a standard care control group. When MI interventions were compared to an alternative intervention such as brief advice, no significant differences were found. Knight et al. (2006) examined MI in physical health care settings and found that although MI interventions showed positive effects on psychological variables, no significant differences were found for other outcomes such as improving knowledge. Knight et al. concluded that the evidence was not currently strong enough to recommend the use of MI in the physical

motivational interviewing in health care

117

health care setting. More high quality randomized control trials of MI are therefore necessary before we can widely apply the technique in health care settings to improve health.

REFERENCES

Grenard, J. L., Ames, S. L., Pentz, M. A. and Sussman, S. (2006) 'Motivational interviewing with adolescents and young adults for drug-related problems', *International Journal of Adolescent Medicine and Health*, 18(1): 53–67.

Hettema, J., Steele, J. and Miller, W. R. (2005) 'Motivational interviewing', *Annual Review of Clinical Psychology*, 1: 91–111.

Knight, K. M., McGowan, L., Dickens, C. and Bundy, C. (2006) 'A systematic review of motivational interviewing in physical health care settings', *British Journal of Health Psychology*, 11(2): 319–32.

Miller, W. R. (1983) 'Motivational interviewing with problem drinkers', *Behavioural Psychotherapy*, 11: 147–72.

Rollnick, S. and Miller, W. R. (1995) 'What is motivational interviewing?', *Behavioural and Cognitive Psychotherapy*, 23: 325–34.

E. D.

Part 5
The Lived Experience of Health and Illness

Stigma and labelling theory

The practical relevance of the sociological construct of 'labelling' has been acknowledged within medical practice since the 1960s. Labelling theory draws attention to the view that the experience of having an illness has both social as well as physical consequences for an individual. This approach, however, is much more concerned with *societal reaction* to the attachment of a chronic disease label than with the physical impact of that illness. Here the notion of the 'symbolic meanings' attached to an illness comes into play. Symbolic meanings are, for sociologists, the shared social connotations and imagery that are associated with particular events and objects and upon which our actions are largely based.

From this perspective, the outcome of the clinical process in which a doctor diagnoses a patient as having a disease involves much more than the identification of a set of physical (or psychological in the case of mental illness) signs and symptoms, it also has social consequences. To diagnose a person as being ill is, from this perspective, to attach a 'label' to that person as someone who has 'deviated' from the social 'norm' of healthiness. Crucial to this approach is the distinction that is drawn between 'sickness' and disease, the former being the social expression (that is, taking on or being given the social role of being 'sick') of the experience of illness. Sickness is thus perceived to be 'a form of deviancy' because it falls outside these social norms in the same way that forms of criminal or anti-social behaviour fall outside the norms of civil society. This understanding draws on the work of Lemert who argued that '[D]eviant behavior is not a property inherent in any particular kind of behavior; it is a property conferred upon that behavior by the people who come into direct or indirect contact with it' (1967). He went on to draw a distinction between 'primary' and 'secondary' deviance. Primary deviance is seen to consist of deviant acts before they are publicly labelled, and has 'only marginal implications for the status and psychic structure of the person concerned'. Secondary deviance is much more significant because it alters a person's self-regard and social roles.

In the case of illness, the primary deviance is the original behaviour of the person when they are feeling unwell unmediated by a societal response.

For the most part, however, sociologists who have utilized labelling theory as an explanation of the social experience of illness have not attempted to account for the original behaviour, but instead have generally concerned themselves with secondary deviance. This is the behaviour that is evoked in individuals by the societal response to their disease label. It is because particular disease labels carry such widely shared public stereotypes (often shared also by health care professionals, because they do not practise in a cultural vacuum) that the behaviour-change characteristic of secondary deviance occurs. For example, the diagnosis of a sexually transmitted disease (STD) or liver cirrhosis (associated with excessive use of alcohol) carries one set of (largely negative) symbolic meanings, while the diagnosis of multiple sclerosis carries a very different set of social meanings. Generally, it is the case that the more socially visible the symptoms, the greater the chance of their becoming social labelling, although this process is also dependent upon the levels of social acceptability of this behaviour.

From this perspective, using the example of mental illness, once an individual has been labelled as having a particular psychiatric disorder (which places a particular emphasis on the power of the medical profession – see Friedson, 1970), they become stripped of their old identity and a new one is ascribed to them. This process leads to the individual internalizing this new identity and associated social status. Individuals are seen to take on the role ('master status') of the psychiatric patient with all its associated set of role expectations. Stigmatization then follows. This has the effect of excluding the labelled 'psychiatric patient' from normal interactions.

The concept of 'stigma', although strongly associated with labelling theory, is concerned less with the social process of labelling disease than with the stigmatizing consequences of that process for an individual, a process that Goffman (1968) described as the 'management of everyday life'. Here, the individual is seen to change their behaviour in accordance with a particular disease label, constituting what he termed 'a self-fulfilling prophecy'. So that when the disease label is attached to a person, the very label itself is seen as having the power, in Goffman's (1968) famous phrase, to 'spoil the sufferer's identity', both personal and social. The social stigma that results from this labelling process derives not only from societal reaction which may produce actual discriminatory experiences (known as 'enacted stigma'), but also the imagined social reaction which can drastically change a person's self-identity ('felt stigma'). The real or imagined experience of stigma can lead onto self-isolation and withdrawal from social life, which further reduces that person's self-confidence. Thus begins a downward spiral of an ever-increasing restriction of social roles and social participation.

Over the years since this model of labelling and associated stigma first developed, a number of critiques have developed which call into question some of its key assumptions, but without necessarily undermining the concept of the 'label' or the process of stigmatization. The first focuses on the way in which the label is used within the model in an overly deterministic manner. That is, the label becomes 'a monkey on the back' that cannot be thrown off by individuals who are then forced to go along with modifying their behaviour in accordance with the social stereotypes that prevail regarding the particular condition. In practice, there are many examples of individuals successfully being able to throw off such labels, one being the Disability Rights movement campaign to raise an awareness of disability less as physical impairment and more in terms of society dis-abling individuals. The model has also been criticized for the uncritical way it assumes that an all-powerful medical profession is in someway complicit in perpetuating the negative connotations of certain disease labels, particularly within psychiatry. Often it is people with a particular condition, or their supporters, who are themselves advocates for a disease label, which they hope will mean less stigma and more understanding and financial support for both research and treatment. The label of Asperger's Syndrome as a disease for example, was received with enthusiasm by those who previously had been thought simply to be strange (Kunitz, 2008).

REFERENCES AND FURTHER READING

Friedson, E. (1970) *Profession of Medicine: A Study in the Sociology of Applied Knowledge*. New York: Dodd, Mead & Company.

Gerhardt, U. (1989) *Ideas about Illness: An Intellectual and Political History of Medical Sociology*. London: Macmillan.

Goffman, E. (1968) *Stigma*. Harmondsworth: Pelican.

Kunitz, S. (2008) 'A case of old wine in re-labeled bottles? A commentary on Aronowitz', *Social Science and Medicine*, 67: 10–13.

Lemert, E. (1967) 'The concept of secondary deviation', in E. Lemert (ed.), *Human Deviance, Social Problems and Social Control*. Englewood Cliffs, NJ: Prentice-Hall.

I. C.

Medicalization

People have and always will encounter aspects of being alive that present problems, cause distress and discomfort. It is just part of the richness of everyday life that not all that we do or experience is pleasant or enjoyable. In previous times if these troubles were particularly unsettling or problematic, then help or assistance may have been sought. Doing so would not have taken someone to their local doctor or physician. Rather, a friend or a local cleric may have been approached to offer advice and support. A distinct trend has been emerging in contemporary society. Those formerly normal travails of life, with which other people in the family or community could have assisted, have increasingly come under the medical gaze. This trend is termed as medicalization.

At its simplest, the concept of 'medicalization' refers to the process and tendency whereby a previously 'normal', albeit potentially distressing, aspect of everyday life and existence becomes a medical problem. Once this redefinition has taken place, medical intervention and treatment are allowed and legitimated, and it is the medical profession that has priority in claiming control and expertise over this new phenomenon. There are many examples of medicalization that can be identified in contemporary society. These range, for example, from emotional states, such as shyness and embarrassment, to physical maladies such as baldness, mental health issues such as overusing alcohol, or to 'natural' biological processes such as pregnancy.

As a sociological concept, medicalization was initially developed in the early 1970s in the work of Zola (1972) and Friedson (1970). In this early material the medical profession was squarely identified as the sole force of medicalization in society. For Zola (1972), this was occurring as a consequence of the medical profession becoming an increasingly powerful social force capable of 'nudging aside, if not incorporating, the more traditional institutions of religion and law'. Ultimately, the medical profession was seeking to control more than its traditional base of 'curing' biological illnesses. Illich (1976) also claimed there were dangers in the expansion of medicine into aspects of life that were hitherto out of bounds to it. He advanced his concept of social iatrogenesis that critiqued modern medicine for over-medicalizing society and making people too willing to admit to illness and weakness.

More contemporary renderings and developments of the concept of medicalization have, however, argued that medicalization is a much more diffuse process than presented in the older material above. Instead of medicalization simply being the activity of an all-powerful medical profession moulding, with its all-conquering medical gaze, and dominating the world to its supposed needs, a wider and disparate range of processes, agents and social trends all interweave, whether intentionally or unintentionally, to medicalize certain elements of people's lives that may cause them or others distress.

One interesting process is that the activity of social movements formed by marginalized groups in society who actively campaign for an aspect of human experience is to be seen as a medical problem. Here medicalization is the outcome not of a 'top-down' process of powerful professionals located in powerful institutions but a 'bottom-up' process whereby people with a shared experience actively seek to have their experiences reinterpreted as a medical issue. The hope here is that by doing so they will find help for their condition and it will redress or lessen social stigma.

A useful example of this is alcohol dependency. Traditionally alcohol misuse was regarded as very firmly being the sign of a weak and immoral individual. Consequently, it was the church that was regarded as being the legitimate body that was concerned with tackling and 'curing' alcohol misuse in society. Prayer, temperance and becoming more godly were the preferred means of dealing with those who drank too much. Groups such as Alcoholics Anonymous, for example, were central in redefining drinking to levels that had the potential to cause problems for the individual, their family and wider society as a health problem.

More recently, Conrad (2007) has further refined the concept and identified three new 'engines of medicalization'. The medical profession still occupies an important role in medicalization, according to Conrad, particularly in its gatekeeper role to resources, but its overall power is vastly diminished. The first engine is bio-technology and the power of pharmaceutical companies. The increasing power of pharmaceutical companies allows them to circumvent doctors and the medical profession. Using their economic power to directly market their products to both doctors and (more so in the United States than in Europe) the general public, they have transformed commonplace concerns into medical issues. An obvious example is Viagra. It has ceased to be purely a treatment for older men with some underlying biological cause of impotence. Clever marketing by the drug companies has led to the lowering of the threshold of what constitutes a sexual health problem. The type of person who may wish to take the drug has now been expanded to include men of all ages, who have no biological issues with impotence, but rather have 'erectile dysfunction', a condition whereby temporary loss of erection is experienced as opposed to the long-term inability of impotence.

The rise of consumer culture acts as another engine of medicalization. Consumers who have the economic resources though appropriate health insurance or personal wealth can exert a considerable influence. Conrad points to how plastic surgery as one example of consumer power has increased with a medicalization of the human body, whereby the various idiosyncrasies and 'imperfections' of the human body are amenable to medical procedures. People as consumers can claim to suffer because their bodies are not what they or society would like them to be. Self-definition is another example of consumer-led medicalization. The proliferation of self-help books and the almost endless power of the internet have furnished people with information with which they believe they can diagnose themselves as having a particular condition. Managed care provides the final engine of medicalization. In the United States managed health care can limit how much is spent on a particular condition, but can also see certain conditions becoming profitable to treat as they become defined as a priority (see **Health care consumerism and patient choice**).

Furedi (2008) goes a step further than Conrad and claims that it is not just the appearance of the above engines that have led to increasing levels of medicalization in society, but rather a wider wholesale socio-cultural shift that has seen a medicalization of everyday life. The development of this trend has been evident from the 1980s onwards where there has been increasingly less opposition to medicalization among the general population and has been further prompted by an increasing emphasis on health in media and everyday discourse. Society, he claims, has become so focused on health that all aspects of human life are seen from a health perspective. Therefore, anything that is difficult or problematic for someone is no longer just part of the vicissitudes of day-to-day living, but rather the result of some form of syndrome or disorder. People themselves are, in effect, now actively involved in the medicalization process, seeking to have whatever they deem to be of distress or concern to them redefined as a medical condition. Shyness, for example, is no longer just a personal characteristic but instead a syndrome that can be cured or its effects lessened by the use of the correct drugs.

Overall, medicalization is a complex concept and social phenomena. The transformation and redefinition of everyday maladies and problems into medical conditions are now animated by a variety of social actors, institutions, and public and private concerns, and no longer just the territorial ambitions of the medical profession.

REFERENCES AND FURTHER READING

Conrad, P. (2007) *The Medicalization of Society: On the Transformation of Human Conditions into Medical Disorders*. Baltimore, MD: Johns Hopkins University Press.
Friedson, E. (1970) *Profession of Medicine*. New York: Dodd Mead.
Furedi, F. (2007) 'Medicalisation in therapy vulture', in D. Wainwright, *A Sociology of Health*. London: Sage.
Illich, I. (1976) *Limits to Medicine*. Harmondsworth: Penguin.
Zola, I. K. (1972) 'Medicine as an institution of social control', *Sociological Review*, 4: 487–504.

C. Y.

Biographical disruption

THE EXPERIENCE OF LIVING WITH A CHRONIC ILLNESS

The experiencing of ill health over a long period of time is very much a feature of twenty-first-century Britain. This phenomenon reflects the massive decline in mortality from infections that was characteristic of the nineteenth and early twentieth centuries, in combination with the increasing percentage of the population who are elderly which has resulted from the increases in life expectancy in the same time period (see **Public health**).

Until the 1970s, sociology had little to say about living with a chronic illness as a social experience, and was largely subsumed under Parson's (1951) conception of the 'sick role' or seen as the concern of other disciplines such as medical science and biology. However, over the past 30 years, the subject of the relationship existing between personal identity and the experience of onset and trajectory of a chronic illness has come to dominate research within medical sociology. As Kelly and Field have argued, '[B]iological facts become social facts because others respond to the person in terms of their physicality. They are also social facts for the individual because the individual sufferer is aware of, and has to take steps to cope with, that physical reality' (1996: 253).

Gerhardt (1989) has identified two distinct approaches to assessing the experience of a chronic illness within medical sociology. First, what she calls a 'crisis model', which is primarily though not exclusively associated with the consequences of labelling and stigma, and where the onset of a chronic illness is seen to irreversibly change the social status of an individual (see **Stigma and labelling theory**). Second, what she calls the 'negotiation model', which focuses upon the emergent nature of the chronic illness experience. Living with a chronic illness is seen as representing a potential loss of self, in which the individual struggles to maintain 'normality' over time, and in the face of the uncertainty associated with a degenerative and debilitating chronic illness. This approach therefore places its emphases on 'adaptation' rather than the imposition of a 'deviant identity' as in the stigma and labelling model. The work of Michael Bury and his 'biographical disruption' model are good examples of this 'negotiation' approach to an understanding of the experience.

Michael Bury's sociological work (1988, 1991, 1997) has been particularly concerned with how the 'meanings' of our everyday encounters and interactions change drastically with the onset of a chronic illness, as specific aspects of the condition make themselves felt over time. He describes the experience of chronic illness as leading to a loss of confidence in the body, and from this follows a loss of confidence in social interaction or self-identity, this is the process he terms 'biographical disruption'. The experience of living with a chronic illness and disability is seen as having the effect of cutting across 'the prescriptive patterns of modern social systems'(Bury, 1988: 90). In other words, societal beliefs and the specific social meanings that are attached to the experience of living with a chronic illness strongly influence the societal expectations of what such an individual is able to achieve. Bury goes on to argue that the meaning of an illness for an individual can be seen as operating at two levels:

1 in terms of the problems, social costs and consequences of the disability;
2 in terms of the symbolic significance or connotations that particular illnesses carry.

According to Bury:

> These aspects of meaning in illness are important to an understanding of the strategies that people employ. In essence, the experience of chronic illness involves testing structures of support and risking meanings within the practical constraints of home and work. Relationships do not guarantee particular responses. . . meanings change as they are tested and altered as they are put at risk. (1988: 92)

The 'meanings' of chronic illness are not simply personal. They are the result of shared experiences and interactions with others, which may involve 're-negotiating' existing relationships at work (with colleagues and employers) and at home (with a partner and children, friends and close relatives). The chronically ill and disabled person needs to be able to make sense of how their own condition impacts upon their social roles and personal identity before they can begin the process of 'adjusting' to it. This can involve redefining ideas of what is 'good' and 'bad', so that the positive aspects of their lives are emphasized, and the negative impact of the illness lessened. Rather than focusing on the 'problems' of adjustment, Bury emphasizes the potential for an *active coping* response to chronic illness, and here he draws upon Corbin and Strauss's (1991) notion of 'comeback'. This latter concept has two dimensions: first, the 'physical', which refers to the active work (as against a passive response) engaged in by the patient when undergoing medical treatment and rehabilitation, and, second, the 'biographical', the attempt by the patient to reconnect their life prior to diagnosis with the present and future. Bury also employs the term 'coping' in its relativistic sense, that is in terms of different kinds of adaptation rather than the normative use (typically drawn upon by health care professionals) of 'successful' or indeed 'unsuccessful' responses to life with a chronic illness.

More recent work (Green et al., 2007) has attempted to quantitatively operationalize the essentially qualitative concept of biographical disruption. The context of this study is the *life trajectory* (a shorthand for social and economic disruption in the lives of people) of individuals living with multiple sclerosis. A sample of 800 individuals living with MS was compared with a matched sample drawn from the General Household Survey. The results showed that both men and women living with multiple sclerosis are significantly less likely to be employed than those in the general population, and are also significantly more likely to have a 'below average' household income. This finding occurs despite the fact that the study sample were more likely to be in a higher social class and have higher educational levels than people in the general population. The study did correlate employment status with the level of physical disability, but found that even for those whose disability was less severe and who were able to live with assistance, they were still significantly less likely to be employed than the matched sample in the general population. And, although divorce rates were similar between both groups, half the multiple sclerosis sample reported an impact of their condition on their sexual relationship with their partner, which when combined with the stress of care and financial strain, meant that their marital relationship required 'substantial readjustment' in line with the 'negotiation' approach (Green et al., 2007: 533).

REFERENCES AND FURTHER READING

Bury, M. (1988) 'Meanings at risk: the experience of arthritis', in R. Anderson and M. Bury (eds), *Living with Chronic Illness*. London: Unwin Hyman.

Bury, M. (1991) 'The sociology of chronic illness: a review of research and prospects', *Sociology of Health and Illness*, 13(4): 451–68.

Bury, M. (1997) *Health and Illness in a Changing Society*. London: Routledge.

Charmaz, K. (2000) 'Experiencing chronic illness', in G. Albrecht, R. Fitzpatrick and S. Scrimshaw (eds), *The Handbook of Social Studies in Health and Medicine*. London: Sage.

Corbin, J. and Strauss, A. (1991) '"Comeback": the process of overcoming disability', in G. Albrecht and J. Levy (eds), *Advances in Medical Sociology*, vol. 2. Greenwich, CT: JAI Press.

Davey, B (2001) *Experiencing and Explaining Disease*, 4th edn. Buckingham: Open University Press.

Gerhardt. U. (1989) *Ideas about Illness: An Intellectual and Political History of Medical Sociology*. London: Macmillan.

Goffman, E. (1968) *Stigma*. Harmondsworth: Pelican.

Green, G., Todd, J. and Pevalin, D. (2007) 'Biographical disruption associated with multiple sclerosis: using propensity scoring to assess the impact', *Social Science and Medicine*, 65: 524–35.

Kelly, M. (1992) *Colitis*. London: Routledge.

Kelly, M. and Field, D. (1996) 'Medical sociology, chronic illness and the body', *Sociology of Health and Illness*, 18(5): 241–57.

Parsons, T. (1951) *The Social System*. Chicago: Free Press.

Radley, A. (ed.) (1993) *Worlds of Illness: Biographical and Cultural Perspectives*. London: Routledge.

I. C.

Professional–client communication

Professional–client communication is the process of information sharing between client (or patient) and professional. The type and quality of the communication approach can be affected by a number of factors and influence health outcomes, satisfaction and adherence to treatment.

APPROACHES TO COMMUNICATION

The traditional approach to professional–client communication was that of a doctor-centred or directive model. This places the health professional in the role of an authority figure who instructs and directs the passive patient. It was assumed that there was a one-way transfer of knowledge from the expert health professional to the lay person. This type of approach fails to acknowledge that the client/patient will have their own areas of expertise to add to the consultation, e.g. their symptoms and lifestyle. A doctor-centred approach to communication may lead to patients feeling powerless and unable to exercise little control over their own health. An alternative model is the patient-centred or consumerist approach, where the patient makes the decisions about treatment options.

A number of studies have examined these different communication approaches in order to ascertain which produces the best outcome for patients. Savage and Armstrong (1990) randomly allocated participants to either a patient-centred or doctor-centred communication style. For example, participants in the doctor-centred condition were told 'You are suffering from. . .' while the patient-centred condition were asked 'What do you think is wrong?' Participants rated high satisfaction with both styles of communication but, perhaps surprisingly, the doctor-centred style produced the highest ratings. In particular, the doctor-centred directive style suited patients who rarely attended the surgery, had a physical problem, did not receive tests and received a prescription.

Ong et al. (1995) proposed that the two communication approaches should be combined into an integrated doctor-centred and patient-centred method where the health professional leads in their areas of expertise and the patient leads in theirs. This type of approach, a shared decision-making communication approach, increases patient self-efficacy and their sense of control over their own health and is considered the gold standard for health professionals to use. Successful and appropriate communication between professionals and their clients is of vital importance in the health services. Appropriate communication between health professional and patient is crucial in order to achieve an accurate diagnosis, avoid inappropriate investigations, and avoid potential litigation. If communication is unsuccessful, it can lead to increased patient anxiety and distress and poor adherence to treatment regimes. Good quality communication has been linked to better health, shorter hospital stays and quicker recovery.

WHAT INFLUENCES PROFESSIONAL–CLIENT COMMUNICATION?

There are a number of factors that can influence interactions between health professionals and clients. Variations in patients' socio-demographic characteristics such as cultural background, gender and age can all influence the type of communication approach that will be most useful. Health professionals should be aware of the potential impact of cultural factors such as culturally-specific health beliefs, potential privacy or modesty issues and differing perceptions of the status of the health professional. Studies suggest that female patients more readily ask questions, express their concerns and may display more anxiety than male patients. Due to this gender difference, the health professional may need to encourage male patients to disclose any worries they may have and employ strategies so that they feel comfortable asking questions (e.g. encouraging preparation of a question list before the consultation). Age also appears to influence professional–client communication. Older patients tend to prefer their health professional to assume the traditional doctor-centred communication approach. Despite this preference, health professionals should encourage older patients to take an active role in the consultation due to the potential benefits to their health of a shared communication approach. For example, Rodin and Langer (1980) reported improved mental health when institutionalized elderly people were given a degree of control over their lives.

Individual characteristics of professionals will also influence communication in the health setting. For example, the health professional's mood may influence their consultations with clients. Isen et al. (1991) experimentally manipulated medical students' mood then asked them to perform a diagnosis task with hypothetical patient case studies. The positive mood group arrived at the correct diagnosis more quickly and showed a greater interest in the patient's case history. Furthermore, health professionals will, like everyone else, hold a set of personal health beliefs that are likely to be consciously or unconsciously communicated to their patients through the way they present information and discuss topics. For example, when discussing different treatment alternatives, a health professional may present the option as either 'decreasing the chance of death' or 'increasing the chance of survival'. Even a difference this subtle is likely to be due to differing health beliefs and will affect the patient's choice of treatment. Professional's health beliefs are also likely to affect their decision about whether to prescribe treatment to a patient and may help to explain some of the variance reported in prescribing rates (between 15–90 per cent of patients are given a prescription).

Despite the evidence linking improved communication with better health outcomes, some studies suggest that the communication approaches being used with patients fall short of the ideal. A review of the evidence suggests that around 50 per cent of psychosocial and psychiatric problems are missed, 54 per cent of patient problems and 45 per cent of patient concerns are not elicited by the health professional or disclosed by the patient, patients are interrupted on average 18 seconds into the consultation, and patient and health professional fail to agree on the main problem in 50 per cent of visits (Stewart, 1995).

IMPROVING COMMUNICATION

There are a number of simple steps health professionals can employ to improve communication with clients. Maximizing patient understanding is vital to successful communication and treatment. Studies suggest that lay people's understanding of some medical issues is limited. Hadlow and Pitts (1991) asked patients to choose the correct definition for a number of common medical and psychological terms. The correct definitions were applied in only 36 per cent of the terms and understanding of psychological terms was particularly low. It is important for professionals to establish at the start of the consultation exactly what level of patient understanding is present. Understanding can be improved by encouraging patients to prepare a list of the questions they want to be addressed prior to the consultation.

Another way to maximize patient understanding is to improve the client's recall. Ong et al. (2000) examined cancer patients' memory of information given during their medical consultation. Almost 20 per cent of patients did not remember their diagnosis, over 50 per cent did not remember their prognosis, and recall of treatment options and side-effects was low with only around 32–50 per cent of information retained. Ensuring successful recall should be one of the main aims for professional–client communication. Recall can be improved through avoiding the use of medical jargon, giving specific instructions, and considering the primacy–recency effect. The primacy–recency effect results in the first few minutes and the last few minutes of the consultation being retained while the rest is typically forgotten. Health professionals should therefore ensure that important information is summarized and repeated at the end of the consultation. Providing patients with written information to take away is a simple step to improving recall that has been shown to increase knowledge, adherence and improves outcome (Ley and Morris, 1984).

REFERENCES AND FURTHER READING

Hadlow, J., and Pitts, M. (1991) 'The understanding of common health terms by doctors, nurses and patients', *Social Science & Medicine*, 32(2), 193–6.

Isen, A. M., Rosenzweig, A. S. and Young, M. J. (1991) 'The influence of positive affect on clinical problem solving', *Medical Decision Making*, 11: 221–7.

Ley, P. and Morris, L. A. (1984) 'Psychological aspects of written information for patients', in S. Rachman (ed.), *Contributions to Medical Psychology*, vol. 3. Oxford: Pergamon Press.

Ong, L. M. L., De Haes, J. C. J. M., Hoos, A. M. and Lammes, F. B. (1995) 'Doctor–patient communication: a review of the literature', *Social Science and Medicine*, 40(7): 903–18.

Ong., L. M. L., Visser, M. R. M., Lammes, F. B., van der Velden, J., Kuenen, B.C. and de Haes, J. C. J. M. (2000) 'Effect of providing cancer patients with the audiotaped initial consultation on satisfaction, recall and quality of life: a randomized, double-blind study', *Journal of Clinical Oncology*, 18(16), 3052–60.

Rodin, J. and Langer, E. (1980) 'Aging labels: the decline of control and the fall of self-esteem', *Journal of Social Issues*, 36(2):12–29.

Savage, R. and Armstrong, D. (1990) 'Effect of a general practitioner's consulting style on patient's satisfaction: a controlled study', *British Medical Journal*, 301: 968–70. Cited in Ogden, J. (2005) *Heath Psychology: A Textbook*. Maidenhead: Open University Press.

Stewart, M. A. (1995) 'Effective physician–patient communication and health outcomes: a review', *Canadian Medical Association*, 152(9): 1423–33.

E. D.

Pain is the sensory and emotional experience of discomfort which is usually associated with actual or threatened tissue damage or irritation (American Medical Association, 2003). The experience of pain accounts for 80 per cent of physician visits (Lebovits, 2004) and, if long-lasting and severe, can affect general functioning, ability to work, relationships and emotional well-being. Early theories regarded pain as merely a bodily sensation. Descartes viewed pain as a direct response to external painful stimulation, with a direct pathway between the point where pain originates and the brain area responsible for detection of pain. Specificity theory proposed that there are specific sensory receptors each responsible for transmitting warmth, touch or pain. These early theories assumed that pain sensation was an automatic response that was the direct result of tissue damage and that it occurred without any cognitive or psychological influence. They also proposed that pain which is present without any obvious physical damage or cause is 'all in the mind' and distinctly different from 'organic' pain. Evidence to contradict these early theories has meant that today theorists support the involvement of psychological factors in the experience of pain as will now be discussed.

The example of phantom limb pain clearly shows that pain can be present without any known physical cause. This type of pain is sometimes experienced by amputees who report that, after surgery, painful sensation is present in the missing limb. People experiencing this type of pain can continue to do so even after complete healing. There is obviously no physical cause for the pain, as the limb is no longer there, but the sensation of pain from that body part continues. The example of phantom limb pain also shows the inherent variability of the pain experience. Not every amputee experiences this phenomenon, and those who do, report variation in the occurrence and severity. A further example of the individual variability in the pain experience comes from studies examining analgesic use. Beecher (1956) observed both civilians' and soldiers' requests for pain relief in a hospital during the Second World War. Although the two patient groups often had similar levels of tissue damage, 80 per cent of the civilians requested medication while only 25 per cent of soldiers did. This difference may reflect differences in the perceived meaning of pain; for soldiers it may be perceived more positively as it may increase the chance of going home. Many studies have, furthermore, reported the 'placebo effect', where some individuals can report improvement in pain when they have taken a placebo or dummy pill. This demonstrates the powerful effect psychological factors can have on an individual's experience, further contradicting the early models of pain.

One theory that can help to explain these phenomena is the gate-control theory of pain introduced by Melzack and Wall in the 1960s. The model was a departure from the earlier models in that it included a mechanism to account for psychological influences on pain perception. The gate-control theory proposed that a physiological stimulus could produce a pain response but the pathway behind this relationship was complex. The researchers proposed that a 'pain gate' receives messages both from nerve fibres and the brain. The gate is opened by physical messages such as injury or activation of the nerve fibres; emotional factors like depression and anxiety; and by behavioural factors such as attention focused on the pain. When the gate is opened, the individual perceives pain and the more the gate is opened, the greater the perceived pain. The gates closure is also determined by physical, emotional and behavioural factors. Physical factors such as analgesics; emotional factors such as relaxation and optimism; and behavioural influences like distraction all work to close the pain gate. Despite some criticism, the gate-control theory was an improvement over earlier models of pain in a number of ways. It helped to explain individual variations in the pain experience and suggested an interaction between the body and the mind. A further strength of the theory is that it contains a role for the psychosocial influences on the pain experience which will be discussed next.

PSYCHOSOCIAL INFLUENCES ON PAIN

Learning

Research suggests that two forms of learning can play a role in the experience of pain. After repeated pairings of an environment or stimulus with pain, individuals may begin to associate the environment or stimulus with the perception of pain and enhance the pain they feel. If a person learns to associate the dentist with pain, for example, they may come to expect pain at every appointment. This expectation of pain can lead to the person experiencing a greater intensity of pain. A further way that learning may play a role is through reward-learned behaviour. When we feel pain we may display pain behaviours (e.g. grimacing or sighing) which may lead our family and friends and colleagues to offer support (e.g. sympathy, time off work, attention). This support makes us feel better and is rewarding, however, it may also increase our pain perception.

Anxiety/fear

In both experimental and non-experimental studies of pain a correlation exists between anxiety and pain perception. The more anxious a person is, the more likely they are to experience greater pain. In people with a chronic pain condition (pain lasting more than three months), anxiety can increase pain intensity. In individuals experiencing acute pain (sudden pain with shorter duration), successfully treating the pain lessens the anxiety suffered. Fear is also known to increase pain. People who have experienced chronic pain may sometimes understandably develop pain-related fear. This pain-related fear is apparent in the behaviour of some individuals even if they themselves do not recognize it as fear. Individuals with pain-related fear can be reluctant to do certain things or move in a certain way in case it brings on the pain again. Although this may be seen as protective behaviour, it can often be detrimental; this hyper-vigilance means that pain is always on the mind. This increased attentional focus on pain leads to a greater perception of pain as discussed next.

Attention

The degree of attention paid to the painful sensations is central to determining the intensity of the experience. Research investigating experimental pain has shown how helpful distraction can be as a form of pain management. Experimental pain is often induced by asking participants to submerge their arm and hand into a vat of very cold water for varying lengths of time. Studies utilizing this technique have found that individuals who are given a distraction task during the experiment typically report reduced intensity of pain. Further support for the importance of attention comes from research investigating distraction as a technique to help children during painful medical procedures.

Self-efficacy

Self-efficacy refers to an individual's beliefs about their ability to perform a particular behaviour. Pain patients with low self-efficacy may be less likely to follow treatment advice and less likely to self-manage their illness due to their perceived inability. Self-management of illness has been shown to be beneficial to patients' well-being and health, therefore a reduced self-efficacy could have detrimental effects. Researchers suggest that pain-related self-efficacy beliefs are an important determinant of pain experience and pain behaviours.

Treatment/management of pain

Acute pain is generally treated with medication. Chronic pain, where the pain has persisted without obvious biological cause past normal healing time, is treated using a multidimensional approach. Modern treatment for chronic pain applies a bio-psychosocial perspective; one that includes roles for biological, psychological and sociocultural factors in determining pain. Typically chronic pain treatment includes psycho-education to improve patients' self-efficacy to help them manage their own condition. Treatment also involves improving physical functioning and addressing any pain-related fear of movement/exercise. Often treatment includes a goal of decreasing the patients' reliance on drugs through the introduction of alternative means of coping (e.g. relaxation, distraction, increasing social support). Another useful form of treatment for pain conditions that may be used is Cognitive Behavioural Therapy (CBT). CBT utilizes psychological strategies to address underlying emotions and beliefs about pain, along with any unhelpful behaviour.

Our understanding of the nature and causes of pain has improved. We have moved on from believing that pain results as a simple stimulus–response relationship. Modern research acknowledges the importance of psychological factors in the experience of pain and treatment reflects this.

REFERENCES AND FURTHER READING

American Medical Association (2003) *American Medical Association Complete Medical Encyclopedia*. New York: Random House.

Beecher, H. K. (1956) 'Relationship of significance of wound to the pain experienced', *Journal of the American Medical Association*, 161: 1609–13.

Lebovits, A. (2004) 'Pain', in E. P. Sarrafino (ed.), *Health Psychology Biopsychosocial Interactions*, 6th edn. New York: John Wiley & Sons.

Melzack, R. and Wall, P. D. (1965) 'Pain mechanisms: a new theory', *Science*, 150: 971–9.

E. D.

key concepts in
health studies

Illness narratives

The concept of an 'illness narrative' represents the process by which people with a chronic illness construct and make sense of their past, present and future. As the 'narrative' element of the concept implies, this concept is about story telling, personal biography, interpreting and reinterpreting changes that speaks to the relationship of self, body and society and how chronically ill people create and communicate a presentation of self that is meaningful for both them and for wider society.

As Jewson (1976) notes, prior to the development of modern medicine an essential part of any doctor's interaction with a patient was to gather a personal history and to acknowledge their patient's narrative. The physician would attempt to adduce as much detail as possible about the suffering of the person who was seeking their assistance. As a form of interaction between physician and patient, listening to the patient in order to gather as much information as possible had a long historical lineage. In Ancient Greece and Rome, for instance, the ability to listen to a patient was considered to be an essential element of the physician's craft (King, 2006). The practice of involving such verbal accounts of the unwell person related to wider concepts of health in the ancient world and feudal world. In these pre-modern times health was seen not as the simple dysfunction of the physical body. Illness arose, rather, because the whole person, both their mind and their body, was regarded as being 'out-of-balance'. To heal a sick individual required not just intervention on the physical level (often using blood letting and other approaches that do not sit comfortably with the modern mind) but to address disturbance and disruption in the mind and body and to reassert balance in those domains. Doing so necessitated eliciting the person's story and their narrative.

The gathering of intimate information in the sixteenth and seventeenth centuries was also essential in the diagnosis of illness for other reasons too (Bury, 2001). Without the battery of tests and technology at the disposal of the contemporary doctor there was no other way by which insights into a patient's ill health could be made. In the modern period, however, from the mid-nineteenth century onwards, as diagnosis became increasingly informed by scientific and technological methods, the voice of the patient and their narrative and sense of self featured less and less in medical

Illness narratives

139

encounters. It was tests on their blood, or images in X-rays, for example, which indicated the cause of their malaise as opposed to their verbal accounts and interpretations.

This silence of the patient and the denial of their narrative were an enduring feature of early modern medicine as biomedicine asserted its place as the legitimate discourse for all matters connected to health and healing based on its application of rational scientific logic. The perceived illogical and emotional accounts of lay people were seen as irrelevant for the practice of modern scientific medicine (Bury, 2001). Such a situation might have persisted had it not been for changes in wider society and changes in the types of illness that affect contemporary western societies.

The chronic conditions which characterize the disease incidence in twenty-first-century Britain typically involve multiple pathologies and are therefore complex and not easily amenable to effective treatment. The various pharmaceutical and surgical therapies are sometimes of little effect or produce unpleasant and debilitating side-effects. For the person with a chronic condition, the medical aspects of chronic illness are only one (albeit problematic) facet of their lives. The need or the urge to reassert their sense of self and identity can be of much more concern. Life with a chronic illness often continues for long periods of time and existential concerns about who one is and how one can lead a meaningful life are an important focus for people with a chronic illness. Illness narratives are therefore a vital element in this process, the creating, structuring and relating of a sense of self that provides and gives validation of one's identity for both self and society.

Bury's (1991) development of the concept of **biographical disruption** in relation to the experience of chronic illness was a landmark piece of research in developing and focusing attention on illness narratives. Bury's (2001) work has gone on to identify three different forms of illness narratives.

Contingent narratives

Contingent narratives seek to contextualize the chronic illness by identifying the causes of the illness and the possible ramifications that chronic illness may have for family and friends. In Sanders et al.'s (2002) research with older people who experienced painful and disabled joints, for example, the participants interpreted their current ill health with reference to past events in their lives. Their current pain and disability were the outcome and consequence of their life narrative.

Moral narratives

As the name suggests, moral narratives are narratives that seek to establish a sense of worth, legitimacy and to justify the changed circumstances in which they now find themselves. Health has always possessed a moral or normative dimension. Good health, and being fit and active are culturally accepted as being an indication of moral worth, while being ill can still be tainted with ideas of being 'punished' for wrong doing or pursuing a less than wholesome lifestyle. People with a chronic illness are often required to interact with these wider cultural narratives concerning the moral status of illness either by validating their particular situation or by creating a social distance.

Core narratives

Core narratives operate on a deeper cultural level demonstrating the relationship of self to society and refer to how people with chronic illness draw upon prevailing cultural motifs and symbolic resources to communicate their experiences of chronic illness.

There has been subsequent work that alerts us to how gender, age and class introduce nuances and differences into illness narratives. Pound et al. (1998), for example, established that for older people encountering a chronic illness in old age was an expected development in their life narrative. The disruptive consequences of chronic illness were much less as the older people had already anticipated that their life course might be challenged by chronic illness. Seale and Chateris-Black (2008) have identified that class and gender influence how people structure and relate their illness narratives. Men, for example, structure their illness narratives by reference to how their sense of masculinity is destabilized by chronic illness. Men from higher social economic groups are more likely, however, to 'open up' and relate personal experiences of chronic illness and how it has affected them, while men from lower social economic groups are more likely to report their experiences in less personal and in more general terms.

Finally, illness narratives have taken a more pronounced 'literary turn' recently. Narratives are increasingly to be seen in print. Columnists such as Ruth Picardie, Oscar Moore and John Diamond have written about their (ultimately terminal) experiences of having breast cancer, HIV/AIDS and throat cancer in national newspapers respectively, while musician Ben Watt detailed his experiences of auto-immune disease in his autobiography. The internet has also opened a sphere of communication where people can 'blog' their accounts of chronic illness or interact with others on internet forums and chat rooms.

Illness narratives provide an important and useful conceptual insight into how people make sense of their lives after developing a long-term chronic condition. They also indicate that the maintenance of self is just as important for such people as complying and interacting with the medical side of being chronically ill.

REFERENCES AND FURTHER READING

Bury, M. (1991) 'The sociology of chronic illness: a review of research and prospects', *Sociology of Health and Illness*, 13(4): 451–68.

Bury, M. (2001) 'Illness narratives, fact or fiction?' *Sociology of Health and Illness* 21(3): 263–85.

Jewson, N. D. (1976) 'The disappearance of the sick–man from medical cosmology', 1770–1870. *Sociology*, 10(2): 225–44.

King, H. (2006) *Greek and Roman Medicine*. Bristol: Bristol Classical Press.

Pound, P., Gompertz, P. and Ebrahim, S. (1998) 'Illness in the context of older age: the case of stroke', *Sociology of Health and Illness*, 20(4): 489–506.

Sanders, C., Donovan, J. and Dieppe, P. (2002) 'The significance and consequences of having painful and disabled joints in older age: co-existing accounts of normal and disrupted biographies', *Sociology of Health and Illness*, 24(92): 227–53.

Seale, C. and Chateris-Black, J. (2008) 'The interaction of class and gender in illness narratives', *Sociology*, 42(3): 453–69.

Williams, S. J. (2000) 'Chronic illness as biographical disruption or biographical disruption as chronic illness? Reflections on a core concept', *Sociology of Health and Illness*, 22(1): 40–67.

C. Y.

Adherence

WHAT IS ADHERENCE?

The changing status of the patient or client over the years has resulted in a change of terminology in the area of adherence. Traditionally patient behaviour was discussed in terms of whether they were 'compliant' or not to treatment. Compliance was later seen as being too suggestive of a command given by a powerful health professional to a passive patient. The term 'adherence' has gradually replaced 'compliance' reflecting the change in the health professional–patient relationship. Occasionally the terms 'concordance' and 'adherence' have been used synonymously but in fact they relate to different areas. 'Concordance' describes the patient–professional relationship and consultation process rather than the actual medicine-taking behaviour. Concordance arises through the process of shared decision-making. Defining adherence is further complicated by the differing levels of adherence that are apparent. Can it be said, for example, that a patient missing one pill but taking the rest is non-adherent? Is non-adherence always about not taking medication; can it sometimes be defined as taking too much? How adherence is assessed is also problematic. Some studies rely on indirect self-report measures of adherence to treatment. This method is likely to be open to patients not being frank about their behaviour for fear of disapproval. Direct measures of adherence, such as blood and urine analysis, are invasive and expensive. Despite these conceptual and methodological difficulties, adherence is an important area for research due to the impact on health.

In the 1970s, research was conducted which showed non-adherence to be common. Recent estimates of the prevalence of non-adherence suggest that it may be as high as 35 per cent for prescribed medicine and 85 per cent for behaviour change (Russell, 1999). Non-adherence does not just occur in minor illness. Studies have shown significant levels occur in chronic illnesses such as diabetes and hypertension. The consequences of poor adherence can be costly both to the health of patients and financially to the country. Horwitz et al. (1990) found that heart attack recovery patients with poor adherence were twice as likely to have died at one year follow-up. Non-adherence is also estimated to cost the country hundreds of millions of pounds a year due to the cost of prescriptions being filled but not used and through extra health care demands when treatment is not followed. Understanding what influences adherence behaviour in patients is therefore a worthwhile avenue for research. If we can identify which factors are associated with non-adherence, we can develop methods of improving adherence and thereby improve health.

WHAT INFLUENCES ADHERENCE BEHAVIOUR?

The nature of clinical treatment is likely to affect patient adherence. Patients are less likely to adhere if the treatment plan is complex. This finding may be partly explained by patient understanding which is a key target for health **professional–client communication**. As discussed there, the interaction between health professional and patient can influence adherence to treatment. Ley believed communication to be central to understanding adherence (or, as it was called at the time, compliance). The communication model of compliance (Ley, 1982) is shown in Figure 1.

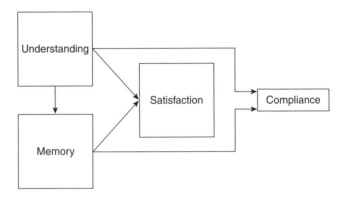

Figure 1   *Communication model of compliance, Ley (1982)*

Ley argued that compliance/adherence can be explained by examining patient satisfaction. Patient compliance is hypothesized to be determined by the interaction between patients' understanding, memory, and satisfaction with consultations. Further influences on adherence will be discussed next.

A recent review (Crumbie, 2002) identified a number of internal and external factors influencing adherence: internal factors such as the patient's age, social background, attitudes, values, emotions, personality, and the type of disease and treatment; external factors such as the impact of health education, the relationship with the health professional, family and friends and social activities also played a role. Hussey and Gilliland (1989) suggest that there are two types of non-adherence: intentional non-adherers and unintentional non-adherers. Unintentional non-adherers do not follow treatment plans because of a chaotic lifestyle or inadequate understanding. Intentional non-adherers, in contrast, do so because they have made a conscious choice influenced by their beliefs. Meichenbaum and Turk (1986) highlighted the types of patient beliefs that were associated with non-adherence. Beliefs such as 'you need to give your body a rest from medicine once in a while otherwise your body becomes dependent/immune to it', and 'how will I know if I'm better if I keep taking the pills?' were associated with non-adherence. Further beliefs about the causes of the illness (e.g. 'my depression is biological, there is nothing I can do') and feelings of resentment at being controlled by drugs also influenced medication-taking behaviour.

Research conducted to examine demographic differences in adherence behaviour found no clear differences for gender, marital status, educational status, socio-economic status or ethnic origin. Age, however, was found to be associated with adherence behaviour, with poorer adherence found in children and the elderly.

Further research suggests a role for psychological factors in treatment behaviour. Bosley et al. (1995) found that non-adherent asthma patients were more likely to be depressed than the adherent group. Perhaps the depressed group felt more hopeless about their illness and more negative about their treatment. Further psychological influences on adherence are suggested by models of health behaviour. The theory of planned behaviour (Azjen, 1991; Azjen and Fishbein, 1980), for example, predicts that adherence to treatment is influenced by the individual's beliefs about the severity of their illness and how susceptible they are to any complications. It further suggests that treatment behaviour will be influenced by the individual's perceived benefits and barriers to treatment.

Patient's recall of treatment advice and instructions is also obviously crucial to ensuring adherence. If an individual has not remembered what their doctor has advised them to do, full adherence is very unlikely. The importance of emphasizing recall during health professional–patient interaction, along with suggestions for improving recall are discussed further on. Further suggestions for improving adherence will be discussed next.

HOW CAN ADHERENCE BE IMPROVED?

Interventions to improve adherence include providing reminders, additional support and supervision by health professionals, and educational counselling. Haynes et al. (2000) conducted a review of studies examining adherence interventions and found that although some combinations of the above were effective; the overall improvement was not great. In addition, the interventions were complex and costly. This finding has led researchers to suggest that the most effective avenue for intervention is to improve communication. Aside from improving communication, the main strategies for improving adherence involve improving the patient's self-efficacy (perceptions about his or her own ability) and empowering the patient.

Buchmann (1997) proposes a number of steps to accomplish this:

- *Make specific enquiries*: careful understanding of the patient's illness and treatment is required in order to develop the best treatment plan.
- *Be benevolent*: A sense that the professional cares about the patient and their problems will increase patient self-esteem.
- *Encourage self-disclosure to gain insight*: Encouraging the patient to elaborate and to give examples will improve professional understanding and patient self-efficacy.
- *Determine the patient's knowledge base*: An understanding of the patient's level of knowledge is important in order both to identify any gaps that may need to be addressed and to acknowledge patient expertise.
- *Determine the patient's commitment*: This will allow the professional to assess what level of patient self-efficacy exists in order to develop plans to improve this if necessary.
- *Maintain an attitude of positive regard*: Appearing shocked, disappointed or annoyed by non-adherence may result in reduced disclosure from the patient and hamper the treatment planning process.
- *Build a sense of personal responsibility*: Taking control for one's own health and treatment is beneficial to patients.
- *Match client needs and wishes*: If treatment options are available, try and match these to the patient's lifestyle and attitudes as far as possible.
- *Use selective positive feedback*: positive feedback promotes a good relationship between professional and client.
- *Attribute endorsed behaviour to a respected secondary group*: Behaviour may be reinforced through discussion of what other respected individuals do.

key concepts in
health studies

REFERENCES

Azjen, I. (1991) 'The theory of planned behaviour', *Organizational Behaviour and Human Decision Processes*, 50: 179–211.

Azjen, I. and Fishbein, M. (1980) *Understanding Attitudes and Predicting Social Behaviour*. Englewood Cliffs, NJ: Prentice-Hall.

Bosley, C. M., Fosbury, J. A. and Cochrane, G. M. (1995) 'The psychosocial factors associated with poor compliance with treatment in asthma', *European Respiratory Journal*, 8: 899–904.

Buchmann, W. F. (1997) 'Adherence: a matter of self-efficacy and power', *Journal of Advanced Nursing*, 26(1): 132–7.

Crumbie, A. (2002) 'Patient professional relationships', in A. Crumbie and J. Lawrence (eds), *Living with a Chronic Condition: A Practitioner's Guide to Providing Care.* Oxford: Elsevier Health Sciences, pp. 3–16.

Haynes, R. B., Montague, P., Oliver, P., McKibbon, K. A., Brouwer, M. C. and Kanani, R. (2000) 'Interventions for helping patients to follow prescriptions for medication', *The Cochrane Database of Systematic Reviews, issue 1.* Oxford: Update Software.

Hussey, L. C. and Gilliland, K. (1989) 'Comliance, low literacy, and locus of control', *The Nursing Clinics of North America*, 24(3): 605–11.

Horwitz, R. I., Viscoli, C. M., Berkman, L., Donaldson, R. M., Horwirz, S. M., Murray, C. J., Ransohoff, D. F. and Sindelar, J. (1990) 'Treatment adherence and risk of death after myocardial infarction', *The Lancet*, 336: 542–5.

Ley, P. (1982) 'Understanding, memory, satisfaction and compliance', *British Journal of Clinical Psychology*, 21: 241–54.

Meichenbaum, D. and Turk, D. C. (1986) *Facilitating Treatment Adherence.* New York: Plenum. Cited in Russell, G. (1999) *Essential Psychology for Nurses and Other Health Professionals.* New York: Routledge.

Russell, G. (1999) *Essential Psychology for Nurses and Other Health Professionals.* New York: Routledge.

E. D.

adherence

Part 6
Health Care Provision

Health care systems

The concept of a 'health care system' is generally normatively (and narrowly) defined as a coordinated system for the management of disease through the provision of clinical health care services (usually coterminous with the boundaries of a national state), rather than as a comprehensive system designed to achieve 'health for all' on the lines of the World Health Organization's definition of health as a 'complete state of physical, mental, and social well-being' (WHO, 1981).

The comparative analysis of health care systems (which usually include some elements of health improvement) generally assesses what have been described as the three key 'functional' dimensions of clinical health care provision as they apply to actually existing health care systems (Freeman, 2000: 1). These dimensions are first, *finance* or the means by which health care systems are paid for; second, forms of health care *provision* or delivery; and, third, the level at which the state intervenes to *regulate* the operation of the health care system (the relationship between these dimensions is schematically represented in Figure 1 overleaf). On this basis, two 'ideal-types' of health care system can be identified as operating in the EU. These are national health service-type models that exist not only in the UK, but also in the Nordic Countries as well as Spain and Italy. And social health insurance-type (SHI) models which exist in France, Germany, the Netherlands and Belgium. However, the use of such 'ideal-types' should be tempered with the understanding that they reflect only a generalized analysis of health care systems, and that national political, economic and cultural priorities mean that changes within health care systems are an on-going process.

HEALTH CARE FINANCE

Within developed countries, three distinct types of organizational arrangements used to finance the health care sector can be found. Funding directly through the state via direct taxation (as in the UK), state-sponsored compulsory social insurance schemes (as in Germany and France), or forms of voluntary private insurance or individualized payment schemes (with the USA being the prime example). Identifying these flows of finance

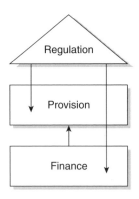

Figure 1   *Three functional dimensions of health care systems*

draws attention to the relative power of the different institutional and political actors within the health care sector in a given country (Crinson, 2009: 97). The most straightforward form of financing is for patients to pay doctors directly for the service that they receive. However, in most developed countries finance is managed by a third party, either the state, not-for-profit organizations, or private insurance companies.

In nearly all EU member states the primary source of financing health is public funding. However, the role played by the state in countries with SHI systems would appear to be of a different order than in those countries with health care systems funded through direct taxation. In these countries, the health care system is not seen as being publicly-owned, in the sense that finance and provision are directly controlled by the state, rather the state is seen as the administrator and guardian of health and welfare structures (Saltman, 2004: 5). This does not mean that the state has a weaker role in health care in countries with SHI systems, just a different role than in countries with direct taxation systems. The state remains the ultimate decision-maker in relation to the determination of the range of health benefits available, the rules for contracting, determining whether there should be mandatory membership, how contributions are calculated, and the degree of discretion in decision-making enjoyed by sickness funds (Busse et al., 2004: 58).

HEALTH CARE PROVISION

The range of care service provision arrangements that exist across the EU member state health care systems may be schematically represented along an organizational axis, from a totally private market through to a universal state scheme. Points along this axis indicate the possible mix of private/public providers in the national health care systems (see Figure 2). Health care provision itself has traditionally been disproportionately focused on in-patient or 'secondary' care. This pattern of provision reflects the historical dominance and autonomy of the medical profession within health care systems and the influence of the biomedical model of disease which focuses on the detailed diagnosis and clinical management of sick patients. Patient access to services and the availability of choice are factors that also reflect the different forms of provision. SHI systems usually offer the choice of doctor or hospital, while those countries which have tax-funded national health services such as Britain utilize a referral system in which the General Practitioner (GP) in Primary Care acts as a 'gatekeeper' limiting patient choice. Nevertheless, it would be a mistake to see the availability of choice as a function of the organization of funding of health care systems alone (Crinson, 2009: 101).

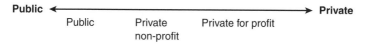

Figure 2 *Health service providers: range of organizational forms*

REGULATION OF HEALTH CARE SYSTEMS

As a conceptual tool, regulation is used in a variety of ways in the literature, but broadly speaking the concept is utilized in order to explain the processes associated with the management of the relationships that exist between the variety of social and organizational actors operating within health care systems. National health care systems are large-scale organizations with complex bureaucratic structures, but patient health care is something that is difficult to effectively and efficiently deliver through such a conventional hierarchical structure. Regulation can provide an alternative or supplementary mechanism for performance management enabling these large organizations to be managed as a network, chain or set of smaller organizations. From this perspective, the NHS would be seen not as one organization but as a network or confederation of about 1,000 organizations – trusts, health authorities, and so on: 'regulatory bodies or agencies are created that take on much of that task of performance management, working to an overall strategy that is set centrally' (Walshe, 2003: 31).

A number of regulatory models can be found in operation in health care systems. In one form, regulation is achieved directly through the imposition of mandatory rules with a strong top-down or command and control role for the state. Regulation can also be achieved through the creation of incentives for competition within a health care market, or it can occur through the building of organizational networks that become mutually dependent upon one another (Saltman, 2002). This range of forms of organizational regulation can be found across European health care systems, and reflect the differing relationships that exist between financing bodies (central government, sickness funds, private insurance companies), service providers (public, not-for-profit agencies, private companies), and service users in these countries. However, at the centre of this regulatory triangle is the medical profession. The demand for health care has traditionally been controlled by the clinical decisions of doctors who decide which services should be made available to patients. In the past two decades, this discretionary power over health care resources has been subject to much greater constraint and scrutiny through the development of new regulatory powers for both national and local health care management structures (see **The role of health professionals**).

REFERENCES AND FURTHER READING

Busse, R., Saltman, R. and Dubois, H. (2004) 'Organization and financing of social insurance systems; current status and recent policy developments', in R. Saltman, R. Busse and J. Figueras (eds), *Social Health Insurance Systems in Western Europe.* Maidenhead: Open University Press, pp. 33–80.

Crinson, I. (2009) *Health Policy: A Critical Perspective.* London: Sage.

Freeman, R. (2000) *The Politics of Health in Europe.* Manchester: Manchester University Press.

Saltman, R. (2002) 'Regulating incentives: the past and present role of the state in health care systems', *Social Science and Medicine*, 54: 1677–84.

Saltman, R. (2004) 'Social health insurance in perspective: the challenge of sustained stability', in R. Saltman, R. Busse and J. Figueras (eds), *Social Health Insurance Systems in Western Europe.* Maidenhead: Open University Press, pp. 3–20.

Walshe, K. (2003) *Regulating Healthcare: A Prescription for Improvement?* Maidenhead: Open University Press.

WHO (World Health Organization) (1981) *Global Health Strategy for All by the Year 2000.* Geneva: WHO.

I. C.

Long-term
health and social
care needs

The concept of 'needs' is a controversial construct if placed in a social context. The conceptualization most cited within the policy literature is derived from Bradshaw's (1972) taxonomy of needs and is set out in a hierarchical form. 'Felt need' is positioned as the base of this hierarchy, and is defined as when people are conscious of their needs but do not explicitly recognize them as such, so they remain largely hidden. Next in the hierarchy is 'expressed needs', this is when an individual becomes aware of their needs and these needs become demands. Next are 'normative needs', which are defined according to health and social care professional norms or standards. Finally, at the very top of the hierarchy are 'comparative needs' which introduces the notion of social justice, i.e. is one social group getting something others are not?

This taxonomy is built upon the premise that needs are socially constructed. By this, it is meant that human social needs are not perceived as universal and transcendental, but rather are a product of a particular society at a particular historical moment. Conceptualizing social needs as being socially constructed is a recognition that an understanding of social and political context is essential. An individual is only able to identify a need for something when the provision to meet that need exists. In the context of the existence of a universal system of welfare state provision of health and social care services such as exists within the UK, it is the *supply* of services that conditions the *demand* for services. Hence, it then becomes possible within social care policy to introduce a set of *eligibility* criteria which can determine what is and what is not a 'need'. This is practicably achievable through the utilization of 'needs assessments' that are now carried out by health and social care professionals in the provision of community care.

However, up until comparatively recently, the term 'Cinderella services' was frequently used to describe the way in which the complex health and social needs of the dependent elderly, people with long-term mental illness, people with physical and learning disabilities, and those living with a long-term mental health problem had been historically marginalized.

However, since the early 1990s, governments of both political persuasions have recognized that this situation has to be addressed, largely because of the increasing proportion of those who are aged 75 and over within the population. Legislation and guidelines have been produced by government in order to coordinate the activities of the NHS and local authorities in order to establish an integrated set of 'community care' services capable of meeting these long-term health and social care needs. One of the most significant changes introduced by the 1990 Community Care Act (which came into operation in 1993) was to place the identification of need for the first time at the centre of the management and service delivery processes. This new emphasis on 'individual needs-based' social planning marked a fundamental policy shift in the delivery of health and social care services in the community.

Further developments in long-term needs-based service delivery came about a decade later in 2001 with the introduction by the New Labour government of a National Service Framework (NSF) for Older People (DoH, 2001). Like all the NSFs, it imposed a series of treatment guideline requirements upon, and regulated the activities of, provider health care organizations. A key requirement of this NSF for Primary Health Care Trusts (PCT) and local authority social service departments was the introduction of a Single Assessment Process (SAP); this was designed to be a tangible representation of the 'interface' of joint health and social needs assessment and care planning for older individuals. The introduction of the SAP moved on the process of client needs assessment that was first introduced in 1993, requiring 'the use of a set of standardized domains of need' in devising an individual care package (DoH, 2001: 31). However, the introduction of standardized assessment of need against which interventions could be planned represented a potential diminution of the judgement of social care professionals. As a recent critique of this evaluative approach noted: 'It is not the level of physical needs *per se* but how these relate to the level of confidence, family support and availability of publicly funded services, as perceived in "the crisis", that determines the need for institutional care' (Taylor and Donnelly, 2006: 825). This commentary points to the necessity of health and social care professionals drawing upon their accumulated experience when assessing the depth of the 'crisis' that has brought the social care needs of an older person to the attention of the local social services; this is not a process that is easily captured in an assessment tool.

In 2006, the government published its policy for social care (*Our Health, Our Care, Our Say: A New Direction For Community Services*,

DoH, 2006) which explicitly defined social care as 'the wide range of services designed to support people to maintain their independence, enable them to play a fuller part in society, protect them in vulnerable situations and manage complex relationships'(DoH, 2006: 3). This new policy to meet long-term health and social care needs marks (in principle) an important shift in the organization and delivery of social care with fewer patients being treated inappropriately in hospital, more services delivered within and near the home with joint health and social care teams assisting people in their daily lives, and more emphasis on preventative care.

In terms of the current numbers, an estimated 1.77 million clients were receiving formal (see **Informal care**) health and social care services in the 'community' (that is, outside of secondary hospital-based in-patient care) in 2007–08, this was unchanged from 2006–07. Of those receiving services, an estimated 1.53 million (87 per cent of all clients) received community-based services, 199,000 received independent sector residential care, 25,000 clients received Local Authority staffed residential care, and 102,000 received nursing care in nursing homes (NHS, 2009). Thus, despite continuing issues of under-resourcing and the building of effective collaboration between local authority social services departments and local NHS organizations, the range and quality of support to meet long-term social needs have undoubtedly improved since 1993. The question remains however, whether future governments will be willing to continue the state provision through general taxation of long-term health and social care services given the demographic fact that the ratio of over-75-year-olds to the rest of the population will continue to rise for many years to come.

REFERENCES AND FURTHER READING

Bradshaw, J. R. (1972) 'The taxonomy of social need', in G. McLachlan (ed.), *Problems and Progress in Medical Care*. Oxford: Oxford University Press.

DoH (Department of Health) (2001) *National Service Framework for Older People in England and Wales*. London: Department of Health.

DoH (Department of Health) (2006) *Our Health, Our Care, Our Say: A New Direction for Community Services*. London: The Stationery Office.

NHS (2009) *Community Care Statistics 2007–08: Referrals, Assessments and Packages of Care for Adults, England*. London: NHS Social Care Information Centre.

Taylor, P. and Donnelly, M. (2006) 'Professional perspectives on decision making about the long-term care of older people', *British Journal of Social Work*, 36: 807–26.

Wanless, D. (2006) *Securing Good Care for Older People: Taking a Long-term View*. London: Kings Fund.

I. C.

Informal care

When examining the whole picture of care provided for people with long-term health and social care needs, an important distinction should be drawn between care that is provided *in* the community (carried out by the Health and Social Services), and care *by* the community. The latter form of care is based primarily upon kinship obligations between members of an immediate family and is generally referred to as 'informal care'. The realities of community care policy (see **Long-term health and social care needs**) in England and Wales (though not Scotland) have meant that informal, essentially unpaid care provision remains predominant. Although the average number of contact hours provided by health and social care professionals to 'clients' receiving 'home care' rose to 9.5 hours per week in 2004 from 7.0 hours in 2000, these figures show the continuing reliance of the social care system on informal carers. 'Home care' is defined as those services which assist the client to function as independently as possible and/or continue to live in their own home. Such services may involve routine household tasks within or outside the home, personal care of the client or respite care in support of the client's regular carers, but they exclude other community-based services such as day care, meals, transport and equipment (NHS, 2009).

It was not until 1985 that a survey of informal carers was carried out by the government (OPCS, 1988). Up until that time, research had focused on the physical and social care needs of those with chronic illnesses and disabilities, while the role of their carers received relatively little focus. The survey revealed that 14 per cent of the population over 16 were 'looking after, or providing some regular service for someone who was sick, elderly or handicapped'. It took a further decade before the Office of National Statistics carried out a much larger survey of informal carers, the findings of which broadly replicated the one carried out in 1985; it found that one adult in eight was providing informal care (ONS, 1998). Government now recognized that much more reliable information was required regarding the numbers of specific caring activities, and so a question was included in the 2001 population census to address this continuing shortfall in knowledge. The 2001 census found that there were 5.2 million unpaid carers (1 in 10 of the population of England and Wales), of which 68 per cent (3.56 million) provided care for up to 19 hours per week, 11 per cent

key concepts in health studies

(0.57 million) provided care for 20 to 49 hours per week, and 21 per cent (1.09 million) provided care for 50 or more hours per week (ONS, 2003)

However, little known about the numbers providing informal care when the first community care policy was introduced in 1990. Although this policy development did for the first time address the issue of who actually performed caring tasks, it also at the same time embedded many of the normative assumptions concerning caring roles that had existed since the inception of the Welfare State.

The first of these assumptions concerned the caring role responsibilities of the family. This assumption in part reflects the widely held and essentially moralistic view that 'problems' arise in meeting the social and health care needs of dependent groups within society because somehow we no longer care for our family members in the way that society did in the past. This view is predicated on an assumption that the role and function of the family have dramatically changed over the past half century with the main change being a shift from the 'extended family' taking responsibility for the care of its sick and elderly members, to the 'nuclear family' of the mid-twentieth century; with the latter seeing many of its caring functions taken over by the state system of welfare. However, this is a simplistic and misinformed reading of the history of the family. It ignores the fact that the major change in the twentieth century was not a shift towards the nuclear family household group, but an absolute decline in the size of families, and a greater geographical dispersion of households containing related people (see **Family and individual well-being**). Crucially, the demographic shift towards people living longer has resulted in an increase in the number of dependent elderly people. Interestingly, as long ago as 1911, 5 per cent of the elderly population were in some type of institutional care, today that proportion is virtually identical (although absolute numbers are very much higher). A second, and related, assumption concerns the role and responsibilities of women in society: the question of what constitutes 'women's work'? In many areas of government health and social policy-making, the implicit assumption is that women are expected to undertake the major role in caring for dependants (including pre-school children, children with disabilities, parents and husbands with disabling illnesses, etc.). However, demographic developments, changes in employment patterns, as well as cultural changes in what is perceived to be the acceptable division of labour within the home between men and women, have meant that the availability of female family members continuing to take on this role in the future cannot be confidently assumed.

There has also been a tendency for policy-makers to assume that caring for dependent relatives is not an issue for ethnic minority communities, reflective of the stereotype of the extended and supportive family network existing among ethnic minorities. Differences in family structure, migration and settlement patterns and socio-economic circumstances have a particularly detrimental effect on the ability of South Asian families to cope with the demands of care-giving in an essentially 'alien' environment (Blackmore, 2000). Moreover, the existence of, and contact with a wider family social support network are no guarantee that help will be freely offered or acceptable to carers and those they care for (Atkin and Ahmed, 2000). One study of the needs of South Asian carers found that the main carer, irrespective of gender, received only limited support both within nuclear and extended households. Although the study found that there was a large potential pool of support for carers within extended families in South Asian communities, in reality, the choice of carer was much more restricted: 'Carers' experiences are affected by the complexity of family dynamics and intergenerational differences in expectations of giving and receiving support' (Katbamna et al., 2004: 402). In addition, it was found that the problems which carers from the South Asian communities face in relation to informal support from within their own families are exacerbated by a lack of support from primary health care services. Female carers generally encountered greater difficulties negotiating and organizing support from formal agencies because of language and communication difficulties, and a lack of knowledge about social and health care service provision. Thus stereotypical assumptions concerning the cultures of ethnic minorities can and do manifest themselves in the perpetuation of inequities in care service provision.

While informal care carried out by lay carers may reduce the financial cost to the state, the costs both to the person being cared for, and to the carer themselves are considerable. Caring can impose a heavy financial (despite state allowances), physical and psychological strain on carers. The carer may have had to give up their own career (unpaid care remains undervalued in society), because it is difficult to combine the demands of paid employment with caring responsibilities. Other outside interests may have had to be curtailed in order to meet the needs of the person with the chronic illness. The physical labour involved in meeting the activities of daily living for a relatively immobile person is also considerable, and likely to be particularly demanding for the carer who is likely to be elderly themselves. Caring relationships between partners and family members are necessarily reciprocal, however, tensions in what were pre-existing relationships (before full-time caring was required) can arise from the changes in role brought about by the increasing dependency of the recipient of care in the relationship. Thus individuals who become physically dependent on their partner may well feel frustration and anger with their condition which they cannot express to their carer in ways that would be possible with a professional carer. In the case of those caring for family members who have a mental health problem, relationships can be strained not just because of the pressure of caring in itself, but because of the ways in which the carers may find themselves stigmatized (by association) because they are seen in some way to be responsible for bringing about the mental health problem in the first place. All these factors can lead to health problems for the carer themselves.

How has government responded to the needs of carers themselves? It was not until 1996 that the first real official recognition of these needs manifested itself in legislation. The Carers (Recognition and Services) Act gave carers (although only those caring for more than 20 hours per week) the right to request an assessment of their own needs. However, the provision of services to all those carers deemed as being in need was never properly resourced and therefore not fully implemented. In 1999, the New Labour government published its national strategy for carers entitled *Caring about Carers* (HMG, 1999). This strategy document represented the outcome of a long consultative process around what was going to become 'a new, substantial policy package that marks a decisive change from what has gone before'. The strategy document set out a number of policy objectives. First, that while unpaid care should be valued, carers should also be supported in combining paid employment with their caring responsibilities in order to prevent their social exclusion. To this end, employers were to be persuaded of the benefits of having 'carer-friendly' employment policies. Second, that carers should be informed and consulted about professional decision-making concerning those they care for. Third, health and social care professionals were to be encouraged to consider the health of carers as part of their responsibilities. Finally, that the support provided to carers should be enhanced in the form of improvements and adaptations to housing, training for carers (especially concerning health and safety within the home), and that there should be provision of regular breaks from caring. In her critical assessment of the Carers Strategy, Liz Lloyd concluded on a positive note by commenting that overall: 'There is innovative and creative thinking in this strategy. It promotes the view of carers as a diverse and widespread group and emphasizes the point that we are all implicated in the way we care for each other' (2000: 148).

Since the establishment of the Carers Strategy, there has been further legislation in support of meeting carers' needs. The 2004 Carers (Equal Opportunities) Act built on the existing legislation to ensure that *all* carers were informed that they were entitled to an assessment of their needs. Many carers continued to remain unaware of their rights despite the hype surrounding the introduction of the Carers Strategy. The Act also placed a duty on councils to consider a carer's outside interests (work, study or leisure) when carrying out a needs assessment. It also sought to promote better joint working between local councils and NHS organizations in order to ensure planning and the provision of services would assist individual carers to continue to care.

REFERENCES AND FURTHER READING

Atkin, K. and Ahmed, W. (2000) 'Family care-giving and chronic illness: how parents cope with a child with sickle cell disorder or thalassaemia', *Health and Social Care in the Community*, 8(1): 57–69.

Blackmore, K. (2000) 'Health and social care needs in minority communities: an over-problematised issue?' *Health and Social Care in the Community*, 8(1): 22–30.

HMG (1999) *Caring about Carers: A National Strategy for Carers.* London: The Stationery Office.

Katbamna, S., Ahmead, W., Bhakta, P., Baker, R. and Parker, G. (2004) 'Do they look after their own? Informal support for South Asian carers', *Health and Social Care in the Community*, 12(5): 398–406.

Lloyd, L. (2000) 'Caring about carers: only half the picture?' *Critical Social Policy*, 20(1): 136–50.

NHS (2009) *Community Care Statistics 2007–08: Referrals, Assessments and Packages of Care for Adults, England.* London: NHS Social Care Information Centre.

ONS (1998) *General Household Survey 1995: Informal Carers: Results of an Independent Study Carried out on Behalf of the Department of Health.* London: The Stationery Office.

ONS (2003) *Census 2001 – Informal Care.* Available at: www. statistics. Gov. uk/census 2001/.

OPCS (1988) *General Household Survey 1985: Informal Carers.* London: HMSO.

I. C.

The role of health professionals

The medical profession has long been seen as the 'paradigmatic profession' within sociological analysis. Studies such as that carried out by Mary Ann Elston have argued that one of the main reasons for the medical profession's pre-eminence within health care systems lies in the fact that it has and remains 'a publicly mandated and state-backed monopolistic supplier of a valued service' (Elston, 1991: 58). The medical profession had already enjoyed a high degree of clinical autonomy in the health care system as it existed before the founding of the NHS, but the establishment and development of this state-funded national health care system (see **Health care systems**) firmly established the position of doctors as 'gatekeepers' to the new health service.

Elston's explanation of the pre-eminence of the medical profession within health care systems follows on from sociological accounts of the process of professionalization. This work draws attention to the role played by the state in the creation and maintenance of monopolistic labour market structures that historically have provided secure institutional arrangements for maintaining the dominant position of the medical profession. Johnson's (1982) historical account examined the trade-off between the profession providing a service (medical service) for the state and in return the state extending the profession's influence and increasing their membership. Doctors were effectively able to negotiate a 'compact' with the state at the foundation of the NHS which Klein (1990) famously described as 'the politics of the double bed', referring to the mutual dependency between the government and the medical profession in the new NHS. The newly created NHS depended upon the medical profession not only for their clinical knowledge and skills to deliver services, but also for their expertise in defining and formulating health care policy. The compact gave doctors control over the everyday allocation of resources, while the role of the state was confined to deciding the level of overall state funding allocated to the NHS. Doctors were then able to determine health need and allocate state health care resources according to their discretionary power; a position the profession continued to occupy for the next half a century.

But how is the autonomy and dominance that has traditionally been enjoyed by the medical profession conceived? In sociological terms, Friedson's (1970) influential work firmly established what was to become known as the 'professional dominance' or 'power approach' model. This approach, strongly influenced by Weberian notions of power, knowledge and status, consciously sought to challenge the prevailing conceptualization of the medical profession as an ethically-bound profession using its expert knowledge rationally and altruistically within a rule-bound organic society (known as the professional 'traits' model). Friedson argued that the power of medicine in modern societies did not derive from a social consensus around its gate-keeping role in legitimating sickness but rested upon two essentially self-serving pillars. The first was its 'autonomy', or the ability of the profession to control its own work activities. The second relates to the control the profession exercises over the work activities of other health care occupations within the division of labour of health care systems, namely its 'dominance'. Elston's (1991) work went onto expand Friedson's notion of autonomy, and identified three distinct categories: 'economic autonomy' as the ability to determine remuneration, 'political autonomy' as the ability to influence policy choices, and 'clinical autonomy' as the profession's right to set its own standards and to control clinical performance. Elston was then able to argue that any decline in one of the forms of medical autonomy does not necessarily effect change in other areas of autonomy and status. Friedson's later work (1994, 2001) on medical dominance follows his assessment of the actual work of doctors within the context of the health care division of labour which identifies what he terms a 'zone of discretion' specific to medical work. At this level, a professional monopoly over certain skills ensures that even rank-and-file doctors are able to maintain a large amount of discretion in their daily work vis-à-vis other health workers. Together, these discretionary powers usually enable doctors to prevent encroachment upon their clinical autonomy, whether that comes from managerialist attempts to monitor their performance or from the nursing or midwifery professions in taking on aspects of work doctors regard as being within their prerogative.

However, while acknowledging the force of Friedson's argument concerning the adaptability of the medical profession to maintain their autonomy in the face of the managerialist reforms to the organization of health care, a point must be reached when it is possible to say that 'things ain't what they used to be'. In relation to the NHS, the point has been reached where an accumulation of challenges to doctors' autonomy has brought about a fundamental shift in the balance of power between the state and the profession. These challenges come from a range of sources within health care systems. First, the threat to clinical autonomy and professional self-regulation enjoyed by doctors following the introduction of new regulatory mechanisms designed to rationalize and more closely manage health care provision. This has had important consequences in terms of a changing balance of authority within health care (see **Health care governance**). Second, the significant loss of public trust and confidence in the profession following a number of high profile medical scandals. Third, the impact of greater demands for patient involvement in their own care reflecting an end to the traditional deference offered to the profession, and frustration with the limited communication concerning treatment. And finally, the consequences of a changing health care division of labour arising out of various technical and rationalization processes occurring with health care systems (Crinson, 2009: 115).

Other health and social care occupations such as nurses, physiotherapists and medical social workers have attempted to emulate this medical model of professionalism: 'However, lacking the doctor's distinctive combination of a highly-regarded body of expertise and skills with a high degree of cohesion and a tradition of forceful political organization, they were unable to achieve the same status' (Langan, 1998: 10). The long-standing pursuit of professional status is arguably the defining feature of the history of modern nursing:

> Nursing has pursued its professional project for over a century, striving to achieve some autonomy and jurisdiction of its own. Its professional milieu is one which the powerful forces of medicine and the hospitals constantly seek to control, or to change the metaphor, they represent the upper and nether millstones between which nursing has always been ground. (Macdonald, 1995: 143)

The origins of nursing's 'professional project' have been attributed to the 'Nightingale movement' of the 1870s which emphasized the female 'virtues' of nursing practice over the development of a more esoteric knowledge base in order to ensure women's control over nursing as an occupation. This strategy succeeded in excluding men from the occupation until the twentieth century by making the indeterminate aspects of nursing impossible for men to acquire. This was the opposite case to that of the medical profession at the time, which excluded women by making it virtually impossible for them to acquire the technical and scientific knowledge necessary to enter the profession. Witz (1992, 1994) has argued that combining the two strategies of exclusion (of men) and usurpation (of some aspects of the medical profession's role) amounted to what is termed a 'dual closure' approach. However, over the course of the next hundred years, nursing's strategy for achieving professional status made very little progress. This was largely due to the continuing dominance and control of the medical profession over the work of nurses, and the 'inaccessibility' of hospital decision-making structures preventing nurses from having a role in effecting organizational change.

The integration of the training of nurses into the system of higher education in the 1990s in the UK did meet the occupation's aim of uncoupling the historical ties between training and the organizational demands of the health care system while also enabling the development of a distinct knowledge base that would 'epistemologically demarcate nursing from medicine' (Allen, 2001: 10). The newly created academic nursing departments began to act as advocates for a 'holistic approach' to care delivery. This holistic approach sought to promote a reformulation of the nurse–patient relationship on a more equal basis, with nurses being educated to promote healing rather than treating patients instrumentally. However, over the last decade there has been widespread and consistent criticism (from NHS managers) concerning the ability of newly-qualified nurses to fit in with the needs of service. It has been argued that this organizational devaluing of holistic care has resulted in a 'professional demoralization' because nurses in practice are not able to actively engage in the work they are trained to value (Dingwall and Allen: 2001: 66).

The attempt to construct a 'new nursing' framework of theory and practice as the basis for the 'professionalizing' of nursing has, therefore, been undermined by the reality of practice, where the care provided by nurses has to be co-ordinated with the needs of a complex organization (Allen, 2001: 14). While historically the 'bundle of tasks' which comprise nursing work has always been fluid, the role that nursing plays as an adjunct to the medical profession in the health care division of labour has remained largely unchanged (Porter, 1996); this is despite not because of the challenges to the self-regulatory autonomy of doctors. The primary driver of these challenges to the historical dominance of the medical profession is the necessity (for the government) to exercise greater control over the efficient use of health resources in the face of rising demands for health care and raised public expectations about the quality of medical interventions. These developments are leading to a reconfiguration of the NHS workforce that will undoubtedly have a fundamental impact on the role of the health care professional in the future (Crinson, 2008: 264).

REFERENCES AND FURTHER READING

Allen, D. (2001) *The Changing Shape of Nursing Practice*. London: Routledge.

Crinson, I. (2008) 'The health professions', in G. Scambler (ed.), *Sociology as Applied to Medicine*, 6th edn. London: Elsevier, pp. 252–64.

Crinson, I. (2009) *Health Policy: A Critical Perspective*. London: Sage.

Dingwall, R. and Allen, D. (2001) 'The implications of healthcare reforms for the profession of nursing', *Nursing Inquiry*, 8(2): 64–74.

Elston, M.-A. (1991) 'The politics of professional power: medicine in a changing health service', in J. Gabe, M. Calnan and M. Bury (eds), *The Sociology of the Health Service*. London: Routledge, pp. 58–88.

Friedson, E. (1970) *Profession of Medicine*. Chicago: University of Chicago Press.

Friedson, E. (1994) *Professionalism Reborn*. Cambridge: Polity Press.

Friedson, E. (2001) *Professionalism: The Third Logic*. Cambridge: Polity Press.

Johnson, T. (1982) 'The state and the professions: peculiarities of the British', in A. Giddens and G. MacKenzie (eds), *Social Class and the Division of Labour*. Cambridge. Cambridge University Press.

Klein. (1990) 'The state and the profession: the politics of the double bed', *British Medical Journal*, 301: 700–02.

Langan, R. (1998) 'Rationing health care', in M. Langan (ed.), *Welfare: Needs, Rights and Risks*. London: Routledge, pp. 35–80.

Macdonald, K. (1995) *The Sociology of the Professions*. London: Sage.

Porter, S. (1996) 'Breaking the boundaries between nursing and sociology: a critical realist ethnography of the theory–practice gap', *Journal of Advanced Nursing*, 24: 413–20.

Witz, A. (1992) *Professions and Patriarchy*. London: Routledge.

Witz, A. (1994) 'The challenge of nursing', in J, Gabe, D. Kelleher and G. Williams (eds), *Challenging Medicine*. London: Routledge, pp. 23–45.

I. C.

the role of health professionals

167

Health care governance

The concept 'governance' is multi-layered, complex and difficult to define, but at its simplest it is the way 'in which organizations and the people working in them relate to each other' (Davies et al., 2005: 21). The notion of governance is essentially a conceptualization of the dynamic relationship of authority and control that exists between social structures and social actors. Hence its utilization in attempting to conceptualize the important changes occurring in the way in which society is governed, and in particular the structuring and restructuring of social networks and hierarchies.

It is precisely because of this concern with contextually bound relational social practices that different modes or types of governance are identified within the literature. These can include a control and command 'mode' of governance typical of traditional forms of top-down hierarchical government or organizational bureaucracies (this type can also be seen as a form of regulation – see below for discussion on this point). Second, a mode of governance that focuses on building a shared value system or frame of reference within an organization or service. This is a form of 'self-governance', examples of which might include self-managing teams, work incentives based on mutuality, and a shared professional or occupational identity. Third, a contractual mode based upon an inducement–contribution exchange between different parties, typically found in market-led services. And, fourth, an emergent form of governance that Newman (2001) has described as 'network governance'. Examples of this form of governance can increasingly be found within the public services and involve negotiation across organizational boundaries to achieve mutually agreed goals, and incentives to work together for these goals, based on reciprocity and trust.

It should be noted that the concepts of 'governance' and 'regulation' are often deployed to describe what outwardly would appear to be similar sets of organizational processes. This can cause some confusion for the unwary. For example, the Department of Health in its NHS reform strategy policy documents, *The NHS Improvement Plan* (DoH, 2004) and *Our Health, Our Care, Our Say* (DoH, 2006), talks about the need to develop a new 'framework' of governance in order to be able to deliver the 'supply-side' reforms of service provision, yet in practice what is being described here is better captured by the concept 'regulation'. In relation to health care, 'regulation' properly describes the *exercise of authority* by the state through the establishment of rules that serve to control and/or incentivize the activities of both social and organizational actors (professions as well as health care trusts) within the system. 'Governance', on the other hand, is an analytical construct that is generally utilized in the context of health care to describe the processes associated with the *relationship of authority* existing between the state, the public (the health service users), and the health and welfare professions entrusted with the implementation of policies that impact upon the lives of these citizens (Crinson, 2009: 112).

Within the NHS, issues of governance are reflected in the way in which the interests and 'social rights of participation' of the three key 'actors' in health care (the state, the professions, and the service users) are balanced one against the other. The role of the state being to resolve the tensions existing between the traditional forms of clinical decision-making autonomy exercised by medical professionals, and the demands for greater public control over their activities. This is the ideal-type relationship of governance often portrayed in policy publications, which conceives of governance in terms of forms of reciprocity existing between participants. However, it should be noted that the state is not a neutral player in this process of governance, having its own sets of interests. New forms of health care governance are reflected in the changing nature of the relationship that exists between the individual responsibility of the citizen-users of health services, and the formal responsibilities of the welfare state towards its citizens. Understanding these processes also requires that we look at the 'intersections and tensions' between the users/citizens, health professions and the state (Kuhlmann, 2006: 8).

Issues of governance within health care are also reflected in the tensions existing between traditional forms of clinical decision-making autonomy and demands for greater public control over the activities of these professional groups. To this end, the New Labour government introduced a new professional accountability and quality assurance structure known as the 'clinical governance framework' on coming to power in 1997. The explicit intention in constructing this framework was not to intervene to overtly regulate the work of doctors, but rather to facilitate the building of 'self-governance' (the second form of governance described above). A key pillar of this clinical governance framework was the promotion of an 'evidence-based practice'. While the medical profession had acknowledged the necessity of moving away from traditional forms of routinized practices, which often lead to unsafe and ineffective patient interventions, integrating best evidence into clinical practice has not always been straightforward. The framework was also constructed with the aim of encouraging doctors to think in wider strategic terms about the efficient use of health care resources. The prevailing government view was that the medical profession had historically only ever been able to conceive of clinical need at the level of the individual patient.

In summary, the concept of governance in relation to health care is concerned to account for the way in which the interests and 'social rights of participation' of the various 'actors' in health care can be balanced, if at all. It is, however, also a concept which 'remains both contested and confused. Nonetheless, the notion of "governance"' serves an important function in going beyond the straightforward notion that only governments govern. It recognises a capacity for getting things done which is not captured in any simple way by the power of government to command' (Davies et al., 2005: 82).

REFERENCES AND FURTHER READING

Crinson, I. (2009) *Health Policy: A Critical Perspective*. London: Sage.

Davies, C., Arnand, P. O., Holloway, J., McConway, K., Newman, J., Story. J. and Thompson, G. (2005) *Links between Governance Incentives and Outcomes: A Review of the Literature*. Report for the National Co-ordinating Centre for NHS Service Delivery and Organisation Research and Development (NCCSDO). Available at: http://www.sdo.nihr.ac.uk/

DoH (Department of Health) (2004) *The NHS Improvement Plan: Putting People at the Heart of Public Service*. Cm 6268. London: The Stationery Office.

DoH (Department of Health) (2006) *Our Health, Our Care, Our Say: A New Direction for Community Services*. London: The Stationery Office.

Gray, A. (2004) 'Governing medicine: an introduction', in A. Gray and S. Harrison (eds), *Governing Medicine: Theory and Practice*. Maidenhead: Open University Press, pp. 5–20.

Kuhlmann, E. (2006) *Modernising Health Care: Reinventing Professions, the State and the Public*. Cambridge: Polity Press.

Newman, J. (2001) *Modernising Governance*. London: Sage.

I. C.

Institutionalization refers to the process whereby an individual can begin to lose their sense of self and identity following admission to a long-stay health or social care institution. The transformation from being independent and active to dependent and passive occurs when the needs of the institution supersede the needs of the individual. As a consequence, the individual can lose their ability to function outside of the institution.

When the 1990 NHS and Community Care Act came into being in the United Kingdom, it marked a radical shift in how people with certain care needs were to be supported by the state. Up until then one of the more common approaches had been to accommodate people in long-term care institutions. Such institutions catered for people with mental health problems or for older people who were deemed to be unable to live on their own (see **Long-term health and social care needs**). A key factor (apart from the apparent financial savings to the state) in this shift from institutional care to supporting people in their own homes was centred on the potential harmful side-effects of institutional care. By the early 1990s, the side-effects of long-term institutional care were widely understood. The process of institutionalization could destabilize the personality, identity and independence of people, leading to a further diminishing of health and the ability to function outside the institution of which they were a part. At worst, a patient or client could become utterly dependent on the institution to meet their basic needs, such as dressing, washing and eating. In some cases, patients could lose their sense of self and retreat into themselves to the extent that they were unable to even communicate with other people. Importantly, it was not any underlying medical or health condition that caused them to behave in this way. It was rather the social environment and the needs of the institution to function as an organization and a bureaucracy that were the root cause. The key concept that assists in explaining and understanding this process is 'institutionalization', and was developed in the 1960s by sociologist Erving Goffman, the main elements of which are outlined below.

Goffman followed the symbolic interactionist approach in sociology. This perspective focuses on the small-scale or micro-level interactions between people, and how various symbols, such as speech, clothing and bodily deportment sustain, construct and transform identity in social encounters when we interact with other people; hence 'symbolic interactionist' or 'symbolic interactionism'. His concept of institutionalization emerged out of his fieldwork in a long-term care home in New York. What he attempted to do there was to explore the effects that being in an institution had on people, both staff and patients. This research and further theoretical elaboration were published in what became the sociological classic *Asylums* in 1968.

Let us start with the observation that all people live their lives in relationship with some form of institution, whether this is the office or factory in which they work, the school or university they attend, or with other social institutions such as the police. There is, however, a very distinct difference between these types of institutions and other types of institution in society. The examples of institutions just mentioned are only partial institutions. This means that they do not dominate and subsume every aspect of life. So, being in the office at work all day may seem dominating but at the end of the working day people are free to go home and to engage in other activities. Goffman identifies, in contrast, what he terms 'total institutions'. These institutions include prisons, monasteries, the army, and, importantly for our purposes here, care homes for the elderly, and facilities for people with chronic mental illness. The critical differences between a total institution and a partial institution are that total institutions take over all aspects of daily life, that there is no 'end-of-the-day' where one goes home. Rather, every activity (for example, sleeping, eating and socializing) takes place within that institution. The institution thus forms a totality of existence for the resident patients or clients.

Institutionalization is a process whereby someone is socialized (Goffman terms this a 'moral career') into being institutionalized. The process involves the loss of the person's sense of self and identity ('mortification of self') that they held prior to entering the institution and replacing it with an identity that suits the needs of the institution ('reorganization of self'). Here we encounter the vitally important role of symbols in the construction of self. Certain symbols, the various props that we use to perform our identities, are removed and can include anything from clothing to the various personal items we have around our homes. These objects are vital for our sense of self as they express both who we want to be and record the narrative of our lives. Losing them makes it harder to maintain that sense of self and identity. Such a loss can happen, for example, when someone has their own clothes removed by the institution to have them replaced by clothing from a communal resource. Or it can happen when someone moves from their own home into an institution leaving the bulk of their possessions behind and only taking a few items with them. Goffman refers to this loss of self as a 'degradation ceremony'.

In addition to the loss of these individual symbols which help to construct individuality, there is also a parallel loss of individual choice and control. Instead of living life according to how one wants to, the individual is immersed into a group. Personal freedom to, for example, choose when to eat or when to go to bed is negated by the demands of an institutional timetable, which in turn orders and structures the patient's or client's day. Goffman refers to this as 'batch' living, a term he borrows from animal husbandry with its connotations of 'herding' people.

It is important to note that Goffman does not maintain that institutions deliberately set out to institutionalize the people in their care. Often it is the unintentional consequence of meeting standards of care that are (paradoxically) designed to protect and provide certain basic standards of living. For example, an institution may be required to provide a certain amount of meals each day but to do so means coordinating members of staff, numbers of patients and various parts of the infrastructure. The meals are made, the patients are fed but this is on a mass scale with the individual's needs being subsumed to the needs of the institution.

One further important point to make is that institutionalization is neither necessarily automatic nor inevitable. Goffman identifies a number of ways which a person can adopt to survive being in an institution. Some of these adaptations can be strategies of resistance where attempts are made to maintain a sense of self:

1. *Colonization*: the patient adapts unenthusiastically to their new situation.
2. *Conversion*: the patient accepts what has happened and becomes institutionalized.
3. *Withdrawal*: as far as possible all contact with other people is minimized.
4. *Intransigence:* the patient resists attempts to convert their behaviour. This resistance can be quite aggressive or not cooperating with the staff in an institution.
5. *Playing it cool:* this adaptation maximizes chances of surviving the institution with much of the sense of self and identity intact. Involves minimizing visibility and staying out of trouble.

(Adapted from Barry and Yuill, 2008)

Prior (1993) has commented that the shift to the community has not necessarily prevented institutionalization occurring. In his study of community care hostels in Northern Ireland, he noted some interesting developments. Even though people were no longer resident in the same building each day as would have previously been the case, nevertheless, he observed that some patients appeared to be exhibiting some aspects of institutionalization. To all extents and purposes, much of the daily lives of the clients were reasonably close to being in an old-style institution. They met and interacted with the same health professionals, lived their lives by a fairly set routine and just because they lived in a building that was officially known as a 'home', they lacked the normal freedoms usually associated with being at home. The institution, in effect, had just been geographically 'extended' and symbolically reordered as opposed to completely transformed.

The concept of institutionalization, therefore, brings to our attention the negative effects of care, indicating what can happen to individuals on entering large-scale institutions where their sense of self is compromised by the needs of the institution.

REFERENCES AND FURTHER READING

Barry, A-M., and Yuill, C. (2008) *Understanding the Sociology of Health: An Introduction.* London: Sage.

Goffman, E. (1968) *Asylums: Essays on the Social Situation of Mental Patients and Other Inmates.* London: Penguin.

Prior, L. (1993)*The Social Organization of Mental Illness.* London: Sage.

C. Y.

Health care consumerism and patient choice

The political discourse of greater 'patient choice' over health care decision-making can be found in the policy agendas of all the major political parties stretching back more than two decades. However, in 2004, the New Labour government finally realized its commitment when it introduced its White Paper, *The NHS Improvement Plan* (DoH, 2004). This goal of achieving patient-centredness in health care delivery is illustrated by the following quote taken from this *Improvement Plan*:

> Rapid access is not enough. To meet today's expectations, patients need to be able to choose from a range of services that best meet their needs and preferences. Between now and 2008, the NHS will be making the changes which enable patients to personalise their care and for those choices to shape the system and the way that it is run. (DoH, 2004: para. 2.9)

It should be noted at this point that 'choice' is a Department of Health policy for England and does not apply to patients who are registered in Northern Ireland, Scotland or Wales.

But what are the origins of this policy development that seeks to place 'patient choice' at the heart of the re-organization of the health service? It has been argued that this 'choice agenda' represents the promotion of a form of ideological populism rather than being a genuine extension of democratic participation in government; 'in the sense that everyone is, or ought to be, entitled to choice' (Clarke and Newman, 2006: 4). To illustrate this point, these authors go on to quote the then Prime Minister, Tony Blair, from a speech made in 2003:

> Extending choice – for the many, not the few – is a key aspect of opening up the system in the way we need. But choice for the many because it boosts equity. It does so for three reasons. First, universal choice gives poorer people the same choices available only to the middle classes. It addresses the current inequity where the better off can switch from poor providers. But

we also need pro-active choice (for example, patient care advisors in the NHS) who can explain the range of options available to each patient. Second, choice sustains social solidarity by keeping better off patients and parents within the NHD and public services. Third, choice puts pressure on low quality providers that poorer people currently rely on. It is choice with equity we are advancing. Choice and consumer power as the route to greater social justice not social division. (Blair, 2003)

Presenting choice in this way fits closely with the ideological discourse known as 'consumerism', which asserts that power resides in the choices exercised by citizens when they purchase and consume goods and services. From this perspective, 'consumer power' is seen as having forged a demand-led market over the past 50 years with important consequences for the efficiency of market corporations. The assertion of 'consumerism' is that the logic of choice that has driven this efficiency in the market will, when transferred to the public sector, bring about improvements to the quality of services as providers seek to respond to the needs of patients as 'customers'; hence the demand for an opening-up of state health and welfare services to the exercise of service user choices (Crinson, 2009: 152).

The NHS Improvement Plan (DoH, 2004) sets-out a four stage strategy for the achievement of a 'patient-led' health service. First, by 'empowering' patients so that they are able to have greater personal control and so be in a position 'to call the shots about the time and place of their care'. Second, the building of a new 'supply' market which will allow patients to choose from any health care provider, yet all treatment procedures will continue to be paid for by the NHS. The third vehicle proposed as a means for the promotion of patient choice was the development of a more extensive electronic patient information system that would more easily facilitate patients to become more actively involved in their own health. Finally, a new organizational payment mechanism termed 'Payment by Results' (PbR) was introduced (it became fully operational in 2008) in order to facilitate the goal of 'money following the patient'. This system, in which the provider of care is paid a fixed amount for each patient procedure it carries out, was designed to raise the quality of services and 'support the exercise of choice by patients' (DoH, 2004: 9–11).

Patients have traditionally been encouraged to 'comply' with the clinical management of their condition recommended by their doctor. The widening patient choice through *The NHS Improvement Plan* has the potential to counter this medical paternalism and encourage a patient-directed focus in medical consultation. However, 'choice' is also a term that is deployed in many different ways in health care. It can refer to the choice of location of treatment, choice of doctor or other health professions, or choice of procedures or other health interventions (Propper et al., 2006). The form of choice introduced following the implementation of *The NHS Improvement Plan* was, however, primarily limited to choice of location of hospital treatment to be offered by GPs to their patients. It is logical to conclude that limiting patient choice to the time and location of hospital appointments on its own is not going to bring about these changes in doctor–patient relationships: 'GPs can still direct patients and control the treatment options that they offer. Patient empowerment cannot happen unless professionals are engaged' (Farrington-Douglas and Allen, 2005: 9).

Implementing the bundle of initiatives (the four strategies described above) aimed to achieve a strategic realignment within the health service, from a 'centrally-directed' service to a patient-led one has not been a straightforward process. The Department of Health has identified, 'the hierarchical traditions of the NHS with professional divides and bureaucratic systems and inflexible processes' (DoH, 2005: para. 4.4) as key constraints. The implicit message behind this statement is that if the goal of patient choice were to be achieved, a new market of providers needed to be allowed to flourish, free from the sectional interests of traditionally dominant groups within the health service.

The promotion of the choice strategy also raises important questions about equity of access and treatment for the NHS of the future. That is, will those patients who are most in need of health care services, the more socially deprived, actually benefit from a greater availability of choice of providers? There is now strong evidence to support the position that inequities in accessing the health service arise from the existence of important social differences in the ability to assert health needs and which in turn reflect differences in familiarity with, and confidence in accessing the health system. Thus inequities 'are compounded by unequal health care-seeking behaviours, which often disadvantage people from poorer, less educated backgrounds' (Farrington-Douglas and Allen, 2005: 6). Nevertheless, this evidence of inequity has been used by Professor Julian Le Grand, who has been an important influence in the development of the government's choice agenda in health care uses to support his essentially pro-market case for wider patient choice. His position is based on the assumption that:

> Empowering all patients to make informed choices about their care could equalize the advantage the middle class patients currently exercise through

their voice and connections. Higher quality and more tailored information delivered to patients at the time they need it could address the 'inverse information law'. (Le Grand et al., 2003: 30)

The choice strategy thus rests heavily on the ability to 'empower' socially disadvantaged patients so that they are able to make informed choices. The consequences of this approach for patients are that with 'empowerment' comes a new set of (individual) responsibilities. However, the question that is posed but rarely answered is what happens to those individuals who do not make appropriate choices about their health needs, and does this represent a system failure or an individual one (Crinson, 2009: 157)?

REFERENCES AND FURTHER READING

Blair, T. (2003) *Fabian Society Annual Lecture: Progress and Justice in the 21ˢᵗ Century*. London: Fabian Society.

Clarke, J. and Newman, J. (2006) 'The People's choice? Citizens, consumers and public services', paper for international workshop, 'Citizenship and Consumption: agency, Norms, Mediations and Spaces', Kings College, Cambridge.

Crinson, I. (2009) *Health Policy: A Critical Perspective*. London: Sage.

DoH (Department of Health) (2004) *The NHS Improvement Plan: Putting People at the Heart of Public Service*, Cm 6268. London: The Stationery Office.

DoH (Department of Health) (2005) *Creating a Patient-led NHS: Delivering the NHS Improvement Plan*. London: Department of Health.

Farrington-Douglas, J. and Allen, J. (2005) *Equitable Choices for Health*. London: IPPR.

Le Grand, J., Dixon, A., Henderson, J., Murray, R. and Poteliakhoff, E. (2003) *Is the NHS Equitable? A Review of the Evidence*. LSE Health and Social Care Discussion Paper No 11. London: London School of Economics and Political Science.

Propper, C., Wilson, D. and Burgess, S. (2006) 'Extending choice in English health care: the implications of the economic evidence', *Journal of Social Policy*, 35(4): 537–57.

I. C.

key concepts in health studies